Department of Health
Welsh Office
Scottish Office Home and Health
DHSS (Northern Ireland

D0247107

Immunisation
against
Infectious
Disease

London HMSO

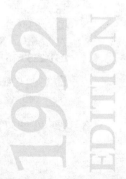

1992
EDITION

First Published 1992

ISBN 0 11 321515 0

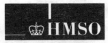

HMSO publications are available from:

HMSO Publications Centre
(Mail, fax and telephone orders only)
PO Box 276, London SW8 5DT
Telephone orders 071-873 9090
General enquiries 071-873 0011
(queuing system in operation for both numbers)
Fax orders 071-873 8200

HMSO Bookshops
49 High Holborn, London WC1V 6HB
(counter service only)
071-873 0011   Fax 071-873 8200
258 Broad Street, Birmingham B1 2HE
021-643 3740   Fax 021-643 6510
Southey House, 33 Wine Street, Bristol BS1 2BQ
0272 264306   Fax 0272 294515
9–21 Princess Street, Manchester M60 8AS
061-834 7201   Fax 061-833 0634
16 Arthur Street, Belfast BT1 4GD
0232 238451   Fax 0232 235401
71 Lothian Road, Edinburgh EH3 9AZ
031-228 4181   Fax 031-229 2734

HMSO's Accredited Agents
(see Yellow Pages)

and through good booksellers

Preface

In the 1990 edition of this Handbook we expressed the hope that it would be updated regularly to keep pace with new developments. Two years later this revision contains details of some important changes and additions, of which perhaps the most noteworthy is the introduction of Haemophilus influenzae b vaccine. (See Chapter 1 "What's new"). In some sections the text has been expanded and in others there are changes which it is hoped will improve clarity and facilitate consistency in interpretation.

The Joint Committee continues to be grateful to everyone involved in immunisation practice for their efforts to ensure that as many children as possible are adequately protected. These efforts are perhaps best reflected in the record low levels of disease notifications and the absence of deaths from measles and pertussis for the last two years and one year respectively. Rubella infections in pregnancy are also at an all time low, reflecting the interruption of transmission from children to susceptible women. The national targets of 90% for immunisation uptake have been attained in England for all vaccines by the second birthday and uptake is showing continuing improvement elsewhere. In the light of these successes, the uptake targets have been raised to 95% by 1995, a perfectly feasible goal as perhaps fewer than 1% of children have genuine contra-indications to immunisation and some health districts have already surpassed 95% for all seven antigens.

There is no room for complacency. The Joint Committee is monitoring the change in age distribution of measles that may require some modification to the immunisation strategy, and is aware of pockets of poor immunisation uptake where unprotected children remain at risk, especially in areas of severe social deprivation and among mobile families. New initiatives are needed to reach these families, or local outbreaks will continue to occur in spite of the favourable picture in the country as a whole.

I should like to record my thanks and that of my colleagues on the Joint Committee to all those who worked on this handbook, but particularly to the editors Dr David Salisbury and Dr Norman Begg, and to Drs Judith Hilton, Jane Leese and Elizabeth Miller and Mrs Maureen Ambler for their efforts in producing this revision.

A G M Campbell MB, FRCP(Edin), DCH
Chairman
Joint Committee on Vaccination and Immunisation

Contents

1   What's New

This edition of Immunisation Against Infectious Disease contains several new sections and there have been many modifications to the information that was in the previous edition. Some of these changes are identified here.

New Vaccines:

From October 1992, **Haemophilus influenzae b (Hib)** vaccine will be given routinely to children along with their primary immunisations. A catch-up campaign is recommended for children who have commenced or completed their primary immunisations and who are under 4 years old. The number of doses required depends on the child's age.

Chapter 8

Hepatitis A vaccine is now available and is recommended for certain travellers and a limited number of high risk groups. For most travellers, immunoglobulin is still recommended.

Chapter 15

Pneumococcal vaccine is recommended for individuals who are at high risk of pneumococcal infection. For some individuals, the risk factors are similar to those for influenza vaccine.

Chapter 14

Typhoid vaccine: Second or subsequent doses of conventional typhoid vaccine can be administered intradermally. Two new typhoid vaccines are now available. A parenteral Vi polysaccharide vaccine requires only a single dose and reactions may be less common than after the whole cell vaccine. The Vi polysaccharide vaccine may produce a sub-optimal response in children under 18 months. A live oral vaccine, taken as one capsule on alternate days for three doses, is suitable for most adults and children over 6 years. Contra-indications are similar to those for other live vaccines. This vaccine contains thermolabile bacteria, so the capsules must remain refrigerated until they are taken.

Chapter 20

New policies:

Pertussis vaccine: There is now a more positive attitude towards immunising children who in the past have been described as having 'problem histories'.

Experience is showing that these children can be immunised without problem, provided that parents are advised about the prevention of pyrexia.

Chapter 5

BCG vaccine: This section has undergone considerable redrafting and now includes details of the disposable head Heaf gun.

Chapter 12

Influenza vaccine: This section now includes advice on the indications for influenza immunisation for young children, along with recommendations on the use of amantadine.

Chapter 13

Hepatitis B vaccine: There has been some modification to the section that describes the risk groups.

Chapter 16

Rabies vaccine: The schedule for the primary course for rabies immunisation has been changed. Three doses are recommended at days 0, 7 and 28.

Chapter 18

Cholera vaccine: Recommendations for the use of cholera vaccine have been severely curtailed. If needed, then the second or subsequent doses can be given intradermally.

Chapter 19

2   Active and passive immunity

2.1   Immunity can be induced, either actively or passively, against a variety of bacterial and viral agents.

2.2   **Active immunity** is induced by using inactivated or attenuated live organisms or their products. Live attenuated vaccines include those for poliomyelitis (OPV), measles, mumps and rubella, and BCG vaccine. Bacterial and viral vaccines such as whooping cough, typhoid and inactivated poliomyelitis (IPV) vaccines contain inactivated organisms. Others such as influenza and pneumococcal vaccine contain immunising components of the organisms; tetanus and diphtheria vaccines contain toxoid – that is, toxins inactivated by treatment with formaldehyde.

2.3   Most vaccines produce their protective effect by stimulating the production of antibodies which are detectable in the serum by laboratory tests. BCG vaccine promotes cell mediated immunity which is demonstrated by a positive tuberculin skin test.

2.4   A first injection of inactivated vaccine or toxoid in a subject without prior exposure to the antigen produces a slow antibody or antitoxin response of predominantly IgM antibody – the primary response. Two injections may be needed to produce such a response. Depending on the potency of the product and time interval, further injections will lead to an accelerated response in which the antibody or antitoxin titre (IgG) rises to a higher level – the secondary response. Following a full course, the antibody or antitoxin levels remain high for months or years, but even if the level of detectable antibody falls, the immune mechanism has been sensitised and a further dose of vaccine reinforces immunity.

2.5   Some inactivated vaccines contain adjuvants, substances which enhance the antibody response. Examples are aluminium phosphate and aluminium hydroxide which are contained in adsorbed diphtheria/tetanus/pertussis vaccine, and adsorbed diphtheria/tetanus vaccine.

2.6   Live attenuated virus vaccines such as measles, rubella and mumps promote a full, long-lasting antibody response after one dose. Live poliomyelitis vaccine (OPV) requires three doses. An important additional effect of poliomyelitis vaccine is the establishment of local immunity in the intestine.

2.7   **Passive immunity** results from the injection of human immunoglobulin (4.10); the protection afforded is immediate but lasts only for a few weeks. There are two types:

     (i)   Human normal immunoglobulin (HNIG) derived from the

pooled plasma of donors and containing antibody to viruses which are currently prevalent in the general population. Examples of the use of HNIG are the protection of immuno-suppressed children exposed to measles, and protection of individuals against hepatitis A.

(ii)   Specific immunoglobulins for tetanus, hepatitis B, rabies and varicella/zoster. These are obtained from the pooled blood of convalescent patients, donors recently immunised with the relevant vaccine, or those who on screening are found to have sufficiently high antibody titres. Each specific immunoglobulin therefore contains antibody at a higher titre than that present in normal immunoglobulin.

2.8   Recommendations for the use of normal and specific immunoglobulins are given in the relevant sections.

3 Introduction

3.1 Consent

(i)   Consent must always be obtained before immunisation.

(ii)   Written consent provides a permanent record, but consent – either written or verbal – is required at the time of each immunisation after the child's fitness and suitability have been established (iv).

(iii)   Consent obtained **before** the occasion upon which a child is brought for immunisation is only an agreement for the child to be included in the immunisation programme.

(iv)   The bringing of a child for immunisation after an invitation to attend for this purpose may be viewed as acceptance that the child may be immunised. When a child is brought for this purpose and fitness and suitability have been established, consent to that immunisation may be implied in the absence of any expressed reservation to the immunisation proceeding at that stage.

(v)   Similarly, the attendance of a child at school on the day that the parent/guardian has been advised that the child will be immunised may also be viewed as acceptance that the child may be immunised, in the absence of any reservation expressed to the contrary. However, because of the parent/ guardian's legal responsibilities in respect of the child's attendance at school, the possibility that immunisation will be offered should be made clear to the parent/guardian.

(vi)   A child under 16 years of age may give consent for immunisation, provided he or she understands fully the benefits and risks involved. However, the child should be encouraged to involve a parent/guardian, if possible, in the decision.

(vii)   Where a child under 16 who fully understands the benefits and risks of the proposed immunisation wishes to refuse the immunisation, that wish should be respected.

(viii)   If a child's fitness and suitability cannot be established, immunisation should be deferred.

3.2   Contraindications

> No child should be denied immunisation without serious thought as
> to the consequences, both for the individual child and for the
> community. Where there is any doubt, advice should be sought from a
> Consultant Paediatrician, Consultant in Public Health Medicine or
> District (Health Board) Immunisation Co-ordinator.

3.2.1

a   If the child is suffering from any acute illness, immunisation should be
postponed until the child has recovered. Minor infections without fever or
systemic upset are not reasons to postpone immunisation.

b   Immunisation should not be carried out in individuals who have a
history of severe local or general reaction to a preceding dose. The following
reactions should be regarded as severe:

> **Local**: an extensive area of redness and swelling which becomes
> indurated and involves most of the antero-lateral surface of the thigh or
> a major part of the circumference of the upper arm.
>
> **General**: fever equal to or more than 39.5°C within 48 hours of vaccine;
> anaphylaxis; bronchospasm; laryngeal oedema; generalised collapse.
> Prolonged unresponsiveness; prolonged inconsolable or high-pitched
> screaming for more than 4 hours; convulsions or encephalopathy
> occurring within 72 hours.

(i)   Immunisation should be postponed if the subject is suffering from any
acute illness. Minor infections in the absence of fever or systemic upset are not
contraindications.

(ii)   Although there is increasing evidence to suggest that rubella vaccine is
not teratogenic (11.3.2), live vaccines should not be administered to pregnant
women because of the theoretical possibility of harm to the fetus. Where there
is a significant risk of exposure, for example to poliomyelitis or yellow fever,
the need for immunisation outweighs any possible risk to the fetus.

(iii)   Live vaccines should not be administered to the following; patients
receiving high-dose corticosteroid (eg for children, prednisolone 2mg per
kilogram per day for more than a week) or immunosuppressive treatment
including general irradiation; those suffering from malignant conditions such
as lymphoma, leukaemia, Hodgkin's disease or other tumours of the
reticuloendothelial system; patients with impaired immunological

mechanisms as for example in hypogammaglobulinaemia. In adults, daily doses in excess of 60mg of prednisolone are associated with significant immunosuppression, although lower doses may be associated with some effect. Under such circumstances, live vaccines such as yellow fever vaccine or BCG should not be used; inactivated vaccines are not dangerous to the recipient but may be ineffective.

(iv)   Individuals with immunosuppression from disease or chemotherapy (eg in remission from acute leukaemia), should not receive live virus vaccines until at least six months after chemotherapy has finished. Such patients and those in (iii) above, should be given an injection of the appropriate preparation of immunoglobulin as soon as possible after exposure to measles or chickenpox (see Sections 10 and 27).

(v)   For individuals treated with systemic corticosteroids at high dose (for children, prednisolone 2mg/kg/day for more than a week; for adults as above), live vaccines should be postponed until at least three months after treatment has stopped. Children on lower daily doses of systemic corticosteroids for less than two weeks, and those on lower doses on alternate day regimens for longer periods, may be given live virus vaccines.

(vi)   Live virus vaccines, with the exception of yellow fever vaccine, should not be given during the three months following injection of immunoglobulin because the immune response may be inhibited. Normal human immunoglobulin obtained from UK residents is unlikely to contain antibody to yellow fever virus which would inactivate the vaccine.

(vii)   For HIV-positive individuals, see 3.4.

In travellers, when time is short and there is a significant risk of exposure to polio, vaccine should be given even if immunoglobulin has been give at any time in the previous three months.

> **Specific contraindications to individual vaccines are given in the relevant sections and must be observed**.

3.2.2   The following conditions are not contraindications to immunisation:-

a   Family history of any adverse reactions following immunisation.
b   Family history of convulsions.
c   Previous history of pertussis, measles, rubella or mumps infection.
d   Prematurity: immunisation should not be postponed.
e   Stable neurological conditions such as cerebral palsy and Down's syndrome.

f   Contact with an infectious disease.

g   Asthma, eczema, hay fever or 'snuffles'.

h   Treatment with antibiotics or locally-acting (eg topical or inhaled) steroids.

i   Child's mother is pregnant.

j   Child being breast fed.

k   History of jaundice after birth.

l   Under a certain weight.

m   Over the age recommended in immunisation schedule.

n   Recent or imminent surgery.

o   'Replacement' corticosteroids

3.2.3   A history of allergy is **not** a contraindication. Hypersensitivity to egg contraindicates influenza vaccine; previous **anaphylactic** reaction to egg contraindicates measles/mumps/rubella, influenza and yellow fever vaccines.

3.2.4   Siblings and close contacts of immunosuppressed children **should** be immunised against measles, mumps and rubella. There is no risk of transmission of virus following immunisation.

3.2.5   Oral poliomyelitis vaccine (OPV) should **not** be given to immunosuppressed children, their siblings or other household contacts. Inactivated poliomyelitis vaccine should be given instead; this should also be given to immunosuppressed adults and their contacts (see 9.3.9).

3.2.6   Homoeopathy: the Council of the Faculty of Homoeopathy strongly supports the programme and has stated that immunisation should be carried out in the normal way using the conventional tested and approved vaccines, in the absence of medical contraindications.

3.3   Special risk groups

3.3.1   Some conditions increase the risk from infectious diseases and children with such conditions should be immunised **as a matter of priority**. These conditions include the following:- asthma, chronic lung and congenital heart diseases, Down's syndrome, antibody-positive to the Human Immunodeficiency Virus (HIV, 3.4), small for dates and born prematurely. This last group should be immunised according to the recommended schedule from two months after birth, irrespective of the extent of prematurity.

3.3.2   If it is necessary to administer more than one live virus vaccine at the same time, they should either be given simultaneously in different sites (unless a combined preparation is used) or be separated by a period of at least three weeks. It is also recommended that a three week interval should be allowed between the administration of live virus vaccines and BCG vaccine (but note 9.5.1).

3.4 Immunisation of individuals with antibody to the Human Immunodeficiency Virus (HIV positive)

3.4.1   HIV positive individuals **with or without symptoms should** receive the following as appropriate;

Live vaccines: **measles: mumps: rubella: polio:**

Inactivated vaccines: **whooping cough: diphtheria: tetanus: polio: typhoid: cholera: hepatitis B: Hib**.

3.4.2   For HIV-positive symptomatic individuals, inactivated polio vaccine (IPV) may be used instead of OPV, at the discretion of the clinician.

3.4.3   HIV-positive individuals should **not** receive **BCG** vaccine; there have been reports of dissemination of BCG in HIV positive individuals.

3.4.4   Yellow fever vaccine should not be given to either symptomatic or asymptomatic HIV-positive individuals since there is as yet insufficient evidence as to the safety of its use. Travellers should be told of this uncertainty and advised not to be immunised unless there are compelling reasons. If such travellers still intend to visit countries where a yellow fever certificate is required for entry, then they should obtain a letter of exemption from a medical practitioner.

3.4.5   No harmful effects have been reported following live attenuated vaccines for **measles, mumps, rubella and polio** in HIV positive individuals who are at increased risk from these diseases. It should be noted that in HIV positive individuals, polio virus may be excreted for longer periods than in normal persons. Contacts of a recently immunised HIV positive individual should be warned of this, and of the need for washing their hands after changing an immunised infant's nappies. For HIV positive contacts of an immunised individual (whether that individual is HIV positive or not) the potential risk of infection is greater than that in normal individuals.

3.4.6   Vaccine efficacy may be reduced in HIV positive individuals. Consideration should be given to the use of normal immunoglobulin for HIV positive individuals after exposure to measles (12.7.1).

3.4.7   For HIV positive individuals exposed to **chickenpox or zoster**, see 27.5.

NB   Some of the above advice differs from that for other immunocompromised patients (3.2).

3.5   Surveillance and reporting of suspected adverse reactions

3.5.1   All vaccines are extensively tested for safety and efficacy before licensing, but careful surveillance must be maintained. This depends on early, complete and accurate reporting of suspected adverse reactions to the Committee on Safety of Medicines, using the yellow card system. **Serious** suspected reactions, including those which are fatal, life-threatening, disabling, incapacitating or which result in hospitalisation **must** be reported; this applies to all serious reactions whether or not such reactions have been previously recognised.

3.5.2   Yellow cards are supplied to general practitioners and pharmacists, and are available from the Committee on Safety of Medicines, 1 Nine Elms Lane, London SW8 5NQ (Tel. 071-273 3000). They are also available as pages of the British National Formulary number 13 (1987) onwards.

4 Immunisation Procedures

> Consent must be obtained (3.1), and suitability for immunisation established.
>
> Doctors and nurses providing immunisation should have received training and be proficient in the appropriate techniques.
>
> Preparations must be made for the management of anaphylaxis and other immediate reactions (see 4.8).

4.1 Preliminary points

4.1.1   These recommendations are based on the current expert advice available to the Joint Committee, although in some circumstances they may differ from that contained in the vaccine manufacturers' data sheets.

(i)   The leaflets supplied with the product and prepared by the manufacturer in consultation with the Licensing Authority should be read.
(ii)   The identity of the vaccine must be checked to ensure the right product is used in the appropriate way on every occasion.
(iii)   The expiry date must be noted.
(iv)   The date of immunisation, title of vaccine and batch number must be recorded on the recipient's record. When two vaccines are given simultaneously, the relevant sites should be recorded to allow any reactions to be related to the causative vaccine.
(v)   The recommended storage conditions must have been observed (see 4.9).

4.2 Reconstitution of vaccines

4.2.1   Freeze dried vaccines must be reconstituted with the diluent supplied and used within the recommended period after reconstitution (see 4.9.6).

4.2.2   Before injection the colour of the product must be checked with that stated by the manufacturer in the package insert. The diluent should be added slowly to avoid frothing. A sterile 1ml syringe with a 21G needle should be used for reconstituting the vaccine, and a small gauge needle for injection (see 4.5).

4.3 Cleaning of skin

4.3.1   If the skin is to be cleaned, alcohol and other disinfecting agents must be allowed to evaporate before injection of vaccine since they can inactivate live vaccine preparations.

4.4 Route of administration

(i)   By mouth

Oral polio vaccine must **never** be injected. OPV should not be allowed to remain at room temperature as this may decrease the potency of the vaccine.

(ii)   Subcutaneous and intramuscular injection

With the exception of BCG and OPV, all vaccines should be given by intramuscular or deep subcutaneous injection. In infants, the antero-lateral aspect of the thigh or upper arm are recommended. If the buttock is used, injection into the upper outer quadrant avoids the risk of sciatic nerve damage. Injection into fatty tissue of the buttock has been shown to reduce the efficacy of hepatitis B vaccine.

(iii)   Intradermal injections

a   Technique

BCG vaccine is **always** given intradermally; rabies, cholera and typhoid vaccines may also be given this way. When giving an intradermal injection, the operator should stretch the skin between the thumb and forefinger of one hand, and with the other slowly insert the needle (size 25G), bevel upwards, for about 2mm into the superficial layers of the dermis, almost parallel with the surface. A raised, blanched bleb showing the tips of the hair follicles is a sign that the injection has been made correctly and its diameter gives a useful indication of the amount that has been injected. Considerable resistance is felt from a correctly given intradermal injection. If this is not felt, and it is suspected that the needle is too deep, it should be removed and reinserted before more vaccine is given. A bleb of 7mm diameter is approximately equivalent to 0.1ml.

b   Suitable sites for intradermal injections

- For BCG the site of injection is over the insertion of the left deltoid muscle; the tip of the shoulder must be avoided because of the increased risk of keloid formation at this site (see 12.19).
- For tuberculin sensitivity tests (Mantoux or Heaf), intradermal injections are given in the middle of the flexor surface of the forearm. This site should not be used for injecting vaccines.

- The use of jet injectors is **not** recommended.
- For intradermal rabies vaccine, the site of injection is behind the posterior border of the distal portion of the deltoid muscle.

4.5   Administration

For deep subcutaneous or intramuscular immunisation in infants, a 23 or 25G needle should be used. For adults, a 23G needle is recommended. Intradermal immunisations should be given with a 25G needle.

4.6   Schedule

4.6.1   **The schedule for primary immunisation with DPT and Hib and polio starts at two months, with an interval of one month between each dose.**[1] This allows completion of the primary course at an earlier age, to provide protection against whooping cough and Hib for the youngest children for whom they are most dangerous. No booster dose of pertussis vaccine or Hib is required; the fourth D/T polio booster continues to be given before school entry.

4.6.2   This accelerated schedule was adopted following recognition that one of the most frequent reasons for low vaccine uptake was the mobility of young families who move out of districts before their children had completed primary courses. This problem was compounded by the variation in schedules between Health Authorities. The new schedule at two, three and four months removes this problem by providing uniformity; starting the programme earlier, and shortening the intervals reduces the opportunities for failing to complete a course.

4.6.3   Studies comparing the antibody levels of diphtheria, pertussis, tetanus and poliomyelitis one year after the third dose showed adequate levels of antibodies for both accelerated and extended schedules.

4.6.4   Studies undertaken to monitor adverse events associated with the accelerated schedule have shown that there are fewer adverse events when compared to the former extended schedules.

4.6.5   Every effort should be made to ensure that **all children are immunised even if they are older than the recommended age-range; no opportunity to immunise should be missed**. The number of doses needed for Hib depends on the child's age (see 8.3). Vaccine is not recommended for those over four years.

---

[1] In some parts of Scotland, the schedule is started at two months and should be completed by six months, with intervals between injections of not less than one month.

4.6.6   When such opportunistic immunisation has been carried out, it must be reported to the Health Authority (HA), NHS Trust, Health Board or Family Health Service Authority (FHSA) as an unscheduled immunisation.

4.6.7   If any course of immunisation is interrupted it should be resumed and completed as soon as possible, but not repeated, except for Hib vaccine when a course must be completed with the same brand of vaccine or recommenced.

4.6.8   The schedule for routine immunisation is given below. Details of procedure for each vaccine are given in the relevant sections and should be consulted.

Vaccine		Age	Notes
D/T/P and polio	1st dose	2 months	
Hib	2nd dose	3 months	Primary Course
	3rd dose	4 months [1]	
Measles/mumps/ rubella (MMR)		12–18 months	Can be given at any age over 12 months
Booster D/T and polio, MMR (if not previously given)		4–5 years	
Rubella		10–14 years	GIRLS ONLY
BCG		10–14 years or infancy	Interval of 3 weeks between BCG and rubella
Booster tetanus and polio		15–18 years	

Children should therefore have received the following vaccines:

By 6 months:	3 doses of DTP, Hib and polio.
By 15 months:	measles/mumps/rubella.
By school entry:	4th DT and polio; measles/mumps/rubella if missed earlier.
Between 10 and 14 years:	BCG; rubella for girls.
Before leaving school:	5th polio and tetanus

[1] In some parts of Scotland, the schedule is started at two months and should be completed by six months, with intervals between injections of not less than one month.

Adults should receive the following vaccines:

Women sero-negative for rubella:	rubella.
Previously unimmunised individuals:	polio, tetanus.
Individuals in high risk groups:	hepatitis B, hepatitis A, influenza.

4.7   Immunisation by nurses

A doctor may delegate responsibility for immunisation to a nurse provided the following conditions are fulfilled:

(i)   The nurse is willing to be professionally accountable for this work.
(ii)   The nurse has received training and is competent in all aspects of immunisation, including the contraindications to specific vaccines.
(iii)   Adequate training has been given in the recognition and treatment of anaphylaxis.

If these conditions are fulfilled and nurses carry out the immunisation in accordance with accepted District Health Authority, NHS Trust or Health Board policy, the Authority/Trust/Board will accept responsibility for immunisation by nurses. Similarly, nurses employed by general practitioners should work to agreed protocols including all the above conditions.

4.8   Anaphylaxis

4.8.1   Recipients of vaccine should remain under observation until they have been seen to be in good health and not be experiencing an immediate adverse reaction. It is not possible to specify an exact length of time.

4.8.2   Anaphylaxis

In the period 1978–89, 118 anaphylactic and anaphylactoid reactions following immunisations were reported to the Committee on Safety of Medicines; no deaths were reported. Furthermore, during this time no deaths from this cause were notified to the Office of Population, Censuses and Surveys (OPCS). During the period approximately 25 million childhood immunisations were given. Anaphylactic reactions are thus very rare, but they are also unexpected and can be fatal. Any individual carrying out immunisation procedures must therefore be able to distinguish between anaphylaxis, convulsions, and fainting. The last is relatively common after immunisation of adults and adolescents; very young children rarely faint and sudden loss of consciousness at this age should be presumed to be an anaphylactic reaction **in the absence of a strong central pulse (ie carotid), which persists during a faint or convulsion**.

4.8.3   The following symptoms may develop:-

a   Pallor, limpness and apnoea are the commonest signs in children.
b   Upper airway obstruction; hoarseness and stridor as a result of angio-oedema involving hypopharynx, epiglottis and larynx.
c   Lower airway obstruction; subjective feelings of retrosternal tightness and dyspnoea with audible expiratory wheeze from bronchospasm.
d   Cardiovascular; sinus tachycardia, profound hypotension in association with tachycardia; severe bradycardia.
e   Skin; characteristic rapid development of urticarial lesions – circumscribed, intensely itchy weals with erythematous raised edges and pale blanched centres.

4.8.4 Management

Such events happen without warning. Adrenaline and appropriate sized oral airways must therefore always be immediately at hand whenever immunisation is given. **All doctors and nurses responsible for immunisation must be familiar with the practical steps necessary to save life following an anaphylactic reaction**.

a   Lie patient in left lateral position. If unconscious, insert airway.
b   Give 1/1000 adrenaline by deep intramuscular injection **unless there is a strong central pulse and the patient's condition is good**. See Table below for dosage.
c   If oxygen is available, give it by face mask.
d   Send for professional assistance. **Never leave the patient alone**.
e   If appropriate, begin cardio-pulmonary resuscitation.
f   Chlorpheniramine maleate (piriton) 2.5-5mg may be given **intravenously**, by appropriately trained individuals. Hydrocortisone (100mg intravenously) may also be given to prevent further deterioration in severely affected cases.
g   If there is no improvement in the patient's condition in ten minutes, repeat the dose of adrenaline up to a maximum of three doses.
h   All cases should be admitted to hospital for observation.
i   The reaction should be reported to the Committee on Safety of Medicines using the yellow card system.

4.8.5   **Adrenaline dosage**:   Adrenaline 1/1000 (1mg/ml)

Adults: 0.5 to 1.0ml repeated as necessary up to a maximum of three doses. The lower dose should be used for the elderly or those of slight build.

Infants and children:

Age	Dose of adrenaline
Less than 1 year	0.05ml
1 year	0.1ml
2 years	0.2ml
3–4 years	0.3ml
5 years	0.4ml
6–10 years	0.5ml

4.9   Storage and disposal of vaccines

4.9.1   Manufacturers' recommendations on storage must be observed and care should be taken to ensure that, on receipt, vaccines are immediately placed under the required storage conditions. Vaccines must not be kept at temperatures below 0°C as freezing can cause the deterioration of the vaccine and breakage of the container.

4.9.2   A pharmacist or other suitably trained person should be nominated for each clinic as being responsible for the safe storage of vaccines, and should work to a written procedure developed to meet local needs. This person should have a designated deputy to cover in times of absence.

4.9.3   A maximum/minimum thermometer should be used in refrigerators where vaccines are stored, irrespective of whether the refrigerator incorporates a temperature indicator dial. Such thermometers may be purchased from reputable laboratory suppliers, some of whom are able to provide a certificate of conformance/calibration (see 4.9.10).

4.9.4   The maximum and minimum temperatures reached should be monitored and recorded regularly and at the least at the beginning of each immunisation session. The written procedure referred to in 4.9.2 should indicate the action to be taken in the event of the temperature going outwith the specified range.

4.9.5   Special care should be taken during defrosting to ensure that the temperature of the vaccine does not exceed the specified range for significant periods of time. An alternative refrigerator or insulated containers should be used for vaccine.

4.9.6   Reconstituted vaccine must be used within the recommended period, varying from one to four hours, according to the manufacturer's instructions. Single dose containers are preferable; once opened, multi-dose vials must not be kept after the end of the session and any vaccine left unused must be discarded.

4.9.7   If vaccines have been dispatched by post, they should not be accepted by the recipient if more than 48 hours have elapsed since posting. The date and time should be clearly marked.

4.9.8   Unused vaccine, spent or partly spent vials should be disposed of safely, preferably by heat inactivation or incineration. Contaminated waste and spillage should be dealt with by heat sterilisation, incineration or chemical disinfection as appropriate. Those providing live vaccines should consult their local Control of Infection Committee about suitable procedures.

4.9.9   Further information and a fact sheet on refrigeration equipment and accessories are available from: Medical Devices Directorate, Product Group 1B, 14 Russell Square, London WC1B 5EP. Tel. No. 071-636 6811 Ext. 3048 or 3059.

4.10   Immunoglobulin (and see under relevant Sections)

4.10.1   All immunoglobulins are prepared from the blood of donors who are negative to hepatitis B (HBsAg) and antibody to human immunodeficiency virus (HIV). The materials are treated to inactivate viruses.

4.10.2   **Human Normal Immunoglobulin (HNIG)**

This is prepared from the pooled plasma of blood donors and contains antibody to measles, varicella, hepatitis A and other viruses which are currently prevalent in the population. Immunoglobulin prepared by Bio Products Laboratory and supplied through PHLS is available in 1.7ml ampoules containing 250mg, and 5ml ampoules containing 750mg. It is given by intramuscular injection. It must be stored at 0–4°C and the expiry date on the packet must be observed. It has a shelf life of three years when correctly stored. Unused portions of an ampoule must be discarded.

4.10.3   Recommendations for the use of HNIG for prophylaxis of measles and hepatitis A are given in 10.7.1 and 15.8 respectively. It is not recommended for prevention of mumps (10.7.2) or rubella (10.7.3).

4.10.4   HNIG may interfere with the immune response to live virus vaccines which should therefore be given at least three weeks before or three months after an injection of HNIG. This does not apply to yellow fever vaccine since HNIG obtained from donors in the UK is unlikely to contain antibody to this virus. For travellers going abroad this interval may not be possible, but in the case of live polio vaccine, this is likely to be a booster dose for which the possible inhibiting effect of HNIG is less important.

4.10.5 Supplies

Central Public Health Laboratory Tel. 081-200 6868
Public Health Laboratories, England and Wales
Blood Transfusion Service, Scotland
Bio Products Laboratory Tel. 081-953 6191
The Laboratories, Belfast City Hospital, Tel. 0232 329341

Immuno. Tel. 0732 458101 (Gammabulin)
Kabivitrum. Tel. 0895 51144 (Kabiglobulin)

4.10.6 Specific Immunoglobulins

These are available for tetanus, hepatitis B, rabies and varicella/zoster. They are prepared from the pooled plasma of blood donors who have a recent history of infection or immunisation, or who on screening are found to have suitably high titres of antibody. Recommendations for their use are given in the relevant Sections:- tetanus (7.3.4 & 7.3.5); hepatitis B (16.10); rabies (18.3.8 (b)); varicella/zoster (27.3 – 27.10).

4.10.7 Supplies

Anti-tetanus immunoglobulin
  Regional Blood Transfusion Centres
  Wellcome. Tel. 0270 583151 (Humotet)
  Scotland: Blood Transfusion Service

Anti-hepatitis B immunoglobulin
  Central Public Health Laboratory Tel. 081-200 6868
  Public Health Laboratories, England and Wales
  Scotland: Blood Transfusion Service (13.8)
  Regional Virus Laboratory, Royal Victoria Hospital, Belfast
  Tel. 0232 240503
  Biotest (UK) Ltd. Tel 021 733 3393

Anti-rabies immunoglobulin
  Central Public Health Laboratory (Virus Reference Laboratory)
  Tel. 081-200 6868
  The Laboratories, Belfast City Hospital, Tel. 0232 329241
  Scotland: Blood Transfusion Service

Anti-Varicella/zoster immunoglobulin
  Communicable Disease Surveillance Centre.
  Tel. 081-200 6868

Public Health Laboratories, England and Wales
Bio Products Laboratory Tel. 081 953 6191
The Laboratories, Belfast City Hospital Tel. 0232 329241
Scotland: Blood Transfusion Service
Biotest (UK) Ltd Tel 021 733 33934.11

Bibliography

Immunisation for the immunosuppressed child.
Campbell A G M.
Arch. Dis. Childhood 1988: 63(2); 113-4.

Human Immunodeficiency Virus infection and routine childhood
immunisation.
von Reyn C F, Clements C J, Mann J M.
The Lancet 1987: ii: 669.

Global Programme on AIDS and Expanded Programme on Immunisation.
Joint WHO/UNICEF statement on early immunisation for HIV-infected
children.
Weekly Epidem. Rec. 1989 No 7. (Feb.17); 48-49.

Immunization of Children infected with Human Immunodeficiency Virus:
supplementary ACIP statement.
MMWR 1988; 37 (12); 181-5.

The efficacy of DPT and oral poliomyelitis immunisation schedules initiated
from birth to 12 weeks of age.
Halsey N, Galazka A.
Bulletin of World Health Organisation 1985: 63 (6); 1151-69.

Durability of immunity to diphtheria, tetanus and poliomyelitis after a three
dose immunisation schedule completed in the first eight months of life.
Jones A E, Johns A, Magrath D I, Melville-Smith M, Sheffield F.
Vaccine 1989: 7; 300-302.

The safe disposal of clinical waste.
Health and Safety Commission: Health Services Advisory Committee, 1982.
HMSO ISBN 0 11 883641 2.

Immunogenicity of combined diphtheria, tetanus and pertussis vaccine given
at 2, 3 and 4 months, versus 3, 5 and 9 months of age.
Booy R, Aitken S J M, Taylor S, Tudor Williams G et al
Lancet 1991: i, 507-510

Diphtheria, pertussis and tetanus vaccination
Cutts F T and Begg N T
The Lancet 1992: 339: 1356

Symptoms following accelerated immunisation schedule with diphtheria,
tetanus and pertussis vaccine
Ramsay M E B, Rao M, Begg N T
BMJ – in press

5   Pertussis

5.1   Introduction

5.1.1   Pertussis is a highly infectious bacterial disease caused by *Bordetella pertussis* and spread by droplet infection; the incubation period is seven to ten days. A case is infectious from seven days after exposure to three weeks after the onset of typical paroxysms. The initial catarrhal stage has an insidious onset and is the most infectious period. An irritating cough gradually becomes paroxysmal, usually within one to two weeks, and often lasts for two to three months. In young infants, the typical "whoop" may never develop and coughing spasms may be followed by periods of apnoea. Pertussis may be complicated by bronchopneumonia, repeated post-tussive vomiting leading to weight loss, and by cerebral hypoxia with a resulting risk of brain damage. Severe complications and deaths occur most commonly in infants under six months of age.

5.1.2   Before the introduction of pertussis immunisation in the 1950's, the average annual number of notifications in England and Wales (E and W) exceeded 100,000. By 1973, when vaccine acceptance was over 80%, annual notifications of pertussis had fallen to around 2,400.

5.1.3   Because of public anxiety about the safety and efficacy of the vaccine, acceptance rates fell to about 30% in 1975 and major epidemics with over 100,000 notified cases followed (in E and W) in 1977/79 and 1981/83. However increased vaccine uptake resulting from the return of public confidence cut short the next epidemic which died away in 1986, well below the levels of the previous two. In 1991, when uptake had risen to 88%, there were only 5207 notifications and the epidemic which had been anticipated failed to materialise.

Figure 5.1 shows the notifications of pertussis for the period 1940 to 1991.

5.1.4   Until the mid 1970's, mortality from pertussis was about one per 1000 notified cases with a higher rate for infants under one year. In 1978 however when there were over 65,000 notifications, (in E and W) only 12 deaths were notified. The actual number of deaths due to pertussis is undoubtedly higher since not all cases in infants are recognised. In 1990, there were six deaths from pertussis, all in infants under four months of age. In 1991, after the immunisation schedule had been accelerated, and the incidence was declining, there were no deaths.

5.1.5   Since the anxieties in the mid 1970's concerning pertussis vaccine, studies have confirmed that a full course of vaccine confers protection in over

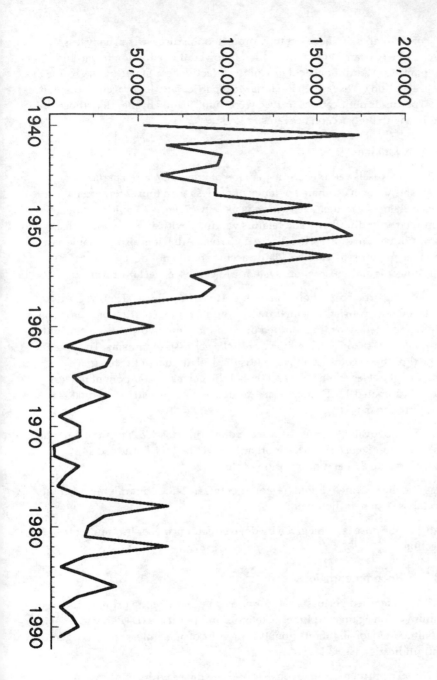

Figure 5.1 Pertussis notifications (E & W) 1940–1991

80% of recipients; in those not fully protected the disease is usually less severe. The two large epidemics which followed the reduction in vaccine acceptance are additional evidence of the effectiveness of pertussis vaccine in the prevention of disease. In Regions with particularly low vaccine acceptance rates, pertussis notifications in 1986 were significantly higher than those in Regions with high acceptance rates.

5.2   Vaccine

5.2.1   Pertussis vaccine is a suspension of killed *Bordetella pertussis* organisms with an estimated potency of not less than four International Units in each 0.5ml of vaccine. The vaccine is usually given as a triple vaccine combined with diphtheria and tetanus vaccines, with an adjuvant such as aluminium hydroxide (DTPer/Vac/Ads, Trivax Ads). It is also available as a monovalent pertussis vaccine. Plain vaccine should not be used as it is less immunogenic and causes more systemic reactions, especially fever.

5.2.2   Adsorbed diphtheria/tetanus/pertussis vaccine (DTPer/Vac/Ads): one 0.5ml dose consists of a mixture in isotonic buffer solution of diphtheria toxoid and tetanus toxoid adsorbed on to aluminium hydroxide gel, together with not more than 20,000 million *Bordetella pertussis* organisms. The potency of the diphtheria component is not less than 30 Iu; that of the tetanus component not less than 60 Iu and that of the pertussis component not less than an estimated 4 Iu. Thiomersal is added as a preservative to a final concentration of 0.01%.

5.2.3   Monovalent pertussis vaccine: one 0.5ml dose contains not more than 20,000 million *Bordetella pertussis* organisms. Thiomersal is added as a preservative to a final concentration of 0.01%.

5.2.4   The vaccines should be stored between 2–8°C, but not frozen. If the vaccine is frozen, it should not be used.

5.2.5   The dose is 0.5ml given by deep subcutaneous or intramuscular injection.

5.3   Recommendations

5.3.1   Adsorbed pertussis vaccine as a component of the primary course of immunisation against diphtheria, tetanus and pertussis (DTPer/Vac/Ads) is recommended for all infants from two months of age, unless there is a genuine contraindication (see 3.2).

5.3.2   The primary course consists of **three doses with an interval of one month between each dose** (see 4.6). If the primary course is interrupted it should be resumed but not repeated, allowing appropriate intervals between the remaining doses.

5.3.3   Monovalent pertussis vaccine can be given when the pertussis component has been omitted from earlier immunisations. Children who have received a full course of immunisation against diphtheria and tetanus should be given three doses of monovalent pertussis vaccine at monthly intervals.

5.3.4   Where the primary course of diphtheria/tetanus immunisation has been started and the parent wishes pertussis vaccine to be added, DTP vaccine may be used for the subsequent doses, followed by monovalent pertussis vaccine at monthly intervals to complete the three doses. Similarly, children presenting for their pre-school diphtheria/tetanus booster who have **not** previously been immunised against pertussis should be given triple vaccine as the first dose, with two subsequent doses of monovalent pertussis vaccine at monthly intervals.

5.3.5   The low uptake of pertussis vaccine from 1975–1985 left a considerable number of unimmunised older children who received DT vaccine only. Such children should be immunised with single antigen pertussis vaccine, both for their own protection and for that of young siblings under the age of immunisation; **there is no upper age limit**.

5.3.6   No reinforcing dose of pertussis vaccine is necessary after a course of three injections.

5.3.7   **Children with problem histories**

When there is a personal or family history of **febrile convulsions**, there is an increased risk of these occurring after pertussis immunisation. In such children, immunisation **is recommended** but advice on the prevention of fever should be given at the time of immunisation.

In a recent British study, children with a family history of epilepsy were immunised with pertussis vaccine without any significant adverse events. These childrens' developmental progress has been normal. In **children with a close family history** (first degree relatives) **of idiopathic epilepsy**, there may be a risk of developing a similar condition, irrespective of vaccine. **Immunisation is recommended for these children.**

Where there is a still evolving neurological problem, immunisation should be deferred until the condition is stable. When there has been a documented history of cerebral damage in the neonatal period, immunisation should be carried out unless there is evidence of an evolving neurological abnormality. If immunisation is to be deferred, then this should be stated on the neonatal discharge summary. **Where there is doubt, appropriate advice should be** sought from a consultant paediatrician, district (Health Board) immunisation co-ordinator or consultant in public health medicine rather than withholding vaccine.

5.3.8   HIV-positive individuals may receive pertussis vaccine in the absence of contraindications given in 3.4.

5.3.9   If pertussis vaccine is contraindicated or refused by parents, then DT/Vac/Ads should be offered.

5.4   Adverse reactions

5.4.1

a   Swelling and redness at the injection site are common (see 3.2.1 b.). A small painless nodule may form at the injection site; this usually disappears and is of no consequence. The incidence of local reactions and pyrexias has been shown to be lower following the accelerated schedule than the previous extended schedule.

b   Crying, screaming and fever may occur after pertussis vaccine in triple vaccine; they may also occur after vaccine which does not contain the pertussis component. Attacks of high pitched screaming, episodes of pallor, cyanosis, limpness, convulsions, as well as local reactions have been reported after both adsorbed DTP and DT vaccines. Both local and systemic reactions were more common after the plain preparations which did not contain adjuvant.

c   More severe neurological conditions, including encephalopathy and prolonged convulsions, resulting in permanent brain damage and death, have been reported after pertussis vaccine. But similar illnesses can develop from a variety of causes in the first year of life in both immunised and unimmunised children and there is no specific test which can identify cases which may be caused by pertussis vaccine. Therefore, no wholly reliable estimate of the risk of such complications due to the vaccine can be made.

d   For these reasons, there has been considerable public and professional anxiety on the safety of pertussis vaccine. In Great Britain, between 1976 and 1979, a total of 1182 children with serious acute neurological illnesses were reported to the National Childhood Encephalopathy Study (NCES). Only 39 of these children had recently had pertussis vaccine and in many of these, the association of the neurological illnesses with immunisation could have occurred by chance. Analysis of the results showed that, after taking this into account, the vaccine may very rarely be associated with the development of severe acute neurological illness in children who were previously apparently normal;

most of these children suffered no apparent harm. **The number of cases in the NCES, even after three years of intensive case finding, was too small to show conclusively whether or not the vaccine can cause permanent brain damage if such damage occurs at all.**

e   In the USA a group of children who had had convulsions or hypotonic-hyporesponsive episodes within 48 hours of DTP were reviewed six to seven years later; there was no evidence of serious neurological damage or intellectual impairment as a result of these episodes. In another American study, while an association was demonstrated between the first febrile convulsion and the scheduled age of pertussis immunisation, no relationship was demonstrated between immunisation and the age of onset of epilepsy.

f   Neurological complications after pertussis disease are considerably more common than after vaccine.

g   Cot deaths (sudden infant death syndrome) occur most commonly during the first year of life and may therefore coincide with the giving of DTP vaccine. However studies have established that this association is temporal rather than causal.

5.4.2   If a febrile convulsion occurs after a dose of triple vaccine, specialist advice should be sought before continuing with any immunisation. Such children are at increased risk of further febrile convulsions following further immunisations. However, these risks can be minimised by appropriate measures to prevent fever and immunisation is recommended.

5.4.3   When pertussis vaccine is genuinely contraindicated, immunisation against diphtheria and tetanus should still be considered.

5.4.4   Severe reactions to pertussis vaccine must be reported to the Committee on Safety of Medicines using the yellow card system.

5.5   Contraindications to pertussis immunisation

5.5.1

a   If the child is suffering from any acute illness, immunisation should be postponed until the child has recovered. Minor infections without fever or systemic upset are not reasons to postpone immunisation.

b   Immunisation should not be carried out in children who have a history of a severe local or general reaction to a preceding dose. Immunisation should be completed with DT vaccine. The following reactions should be regarded as severe:-

Local: an extensive area of redness and swelling which becomes indurated and involves most of the antero-lateral surface of the thigh or a major part of the circumference of the upper arm.

General: fever equal to or more than 39.5°C within 48 hours of vaccine; anaphylaxis; bronchospasm; laryngeal oedema; generalised collapse. Prolonged unresponsiveness; prolonged inconsolable or high-pitched screaming for more than 4 hours; convulsions or encephalopathy occurring within 72 hours.

5.5.2   A personal or family history of allergy is **not** a contraindication to immunisation against pertussis, nor are stable neurological conditions such as cerebral palsy or spina bifida. For other "false contraindications" see (3.2.2).

Where there is doubt, appropriate advice should be sought from a consultant paediatrician, District (Health Board) Immunisation Co-ordinator or Consultant in Public Health Medicine rather than withholding vaccine.

5.7 _ Management of outbreaks

Since a course of three injections is required to protect against pertussis, vaccine cannot be used to control an outbreak.

5.8   Supplies

All pertussis vaccines are manufactured and supplied by Evans Medical Ltd. (Tel. No. 0403 41400).

5.9   Bibliography

Infants and children with convulsions and hypotonic/hyporesponsive episodes following DTP immunisation; follow-up evaluation.
Barraff L J, Shields W D et al.
Pediatrics 1988; 81; 789-794.

Relationship of pertussis immunisation to the onset of neurological disorders: a retrospective epidemiological study.
Shields W D, Nielson C et al.
J. Pediatrics 1988: 81; 801-805.

Vaccination and cot deaths in perspective.
Roberts S C.
Arch. Dis. Child. 1987: 12; 754-9.

DHSS Whooping Cough: Reports from the Committee on Safety of Medicines and the Joint Committee on Vaccination and Immunisation. HMSO 1981.

Severity of notified pertussis.
Miller C L and Fletcher W B.
BMJ 1976, (1), 117-119.

Pertussis immunisation and serious acute neurological illness in children.
Miller D L, Ross E M, Alderslade R, Bellman M H, Rawson N S B.
BMJ 1981: 282; 1595-1599.

Symptoms after primary immunisation with DTP and with DT vaccine.
Pollock T M, Miller E, Mortimer J Y, Smith G.
Lancet 1984: ii; 146-159/

Efficacy of pertussis vaccination in England.
PHLS Epidemiological Research Laboratory and 21 Area Health Authorities.
BMJ 1982: 285; 357-359.

Communicable Disease Report Oct-Dec 1986.
Community Medicine 1987: 9; 176-181.

Immunogenicity of combined diphtheria, tetanus and pertussis vaccine given at 2, 3 and 4 months versus 3, 5 and 9 months of age.
Lancet 1991, i, 507-510
Booy R, Aitken S J M, Taylor S, Tudor-Williams G et al

Pertussis

6   Diphtheria

6.1   Introduction

6.1.1   Diphtheria is an acute infectious disease affecting the upper respiratory tract and occasionally the skin. It is characterised by an inflammatory exudate which forms a greyish membrane in the respiratory tract which may cause obstruction. The incubation period is from two to five days. The disease is communicable for up to four weeks, but carriers may shed organisms for longer. A toxin is produced by diphtheria bacilli which affects particularly myocardium and nervous and adrenal tissues. Spread is by droplet infection and through contact with articles soiled by infected persons (fomites).

6.1.2   Effective protection against the disease is provided by active immunisation. The introduction of immunisation against diphtheria on a national scale in 1940 resulted in a dramatic fall in the number of notified cases and deaths from the disease. In 1940, 46,281 cases with 2,480 deaths were notified, compared with 37 cases and six deaths in 1957. From 1986 to 1991, 13 cases were notified with no deaths.

Figure 6.1 shows the notifications of diphtheria for the period 1940 to 1991.

6.1.3   The disease and the organism have been virtually eliminated from the United Kingdom; the few cases which have occurred in recent years have nearly all been imported. There is thus no possibility now of acquiring natural immunisation from sub-clinical infection. A high immunisation uptake must therefore be maintained in order to protect the population against the possibility of a resurgence of the disease which could follow the introduction of cases or carriers of toxigenic strains from overseas.

6.2   Diphtheria vaccine

6.2.1   Diphtheria immunisation protects by stimulating the production of antitoxin which provides immunity to the effects of the toxin. The immunogen is prepared by treating a cell-free purified preparation of toxin with formaldehyde, thereby converting it into the innocuous diphtheria toxoid. This however is a relatively poor immunogen, and for use as a vaccine it is usually adsorbed onto an adjuvant, either aluminium phosphate or aluminium hydroxide. *Bordetella pertussis* also acts as an effective adjuvant.

6.2.2   The recommended vaccines for immunisation are:
Adsorbed diphtheria/tetanus/pertussis.
Adsorbed diphtheria/tetanus.

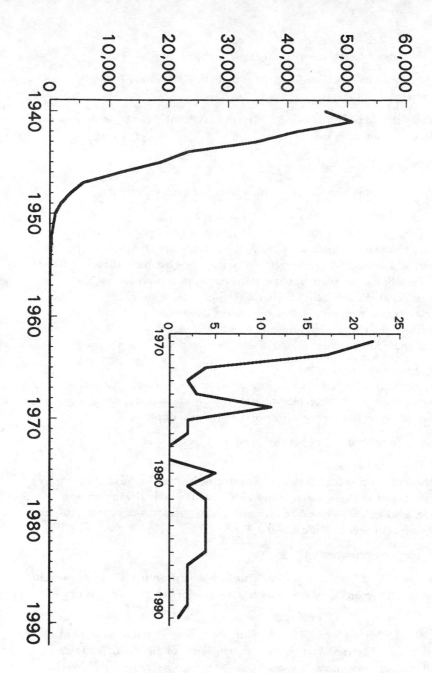

Figure 6.1 Notification of diptheria (E & W) 1940–1991

Adsorbed diphtheria.
Adsorbed low dose diphtheria vaccine for adults.

Plain vaccines are less immunogenic and have no advantage in terms of reaction rates.

Vaccines should be stored at 2–8°C. The dose is 0.5ml given by intramuscular or deep subcutaneous injection.

6.3 Recommendations

6.3.1 For immunisation of infants and children up to ten years.

a Primary immunisation
Diphtheria vaccine as a component of triple vaccine (diphtheria toxoid, tetanus toxoid and *Bordetella pertussis*) is recommended for infants from two months old. **Adsorbed vaccine should be used as it has been shown to cause fewer reactions than plain vaccine**. If the pertussis component is contraindicated, adsorbed diphtheria/tetanus vaccine should be used. **A course of primary immunisation consists of three doses starting at two months with an interval of one month between each dose** (see 4.6). If a course is interrupted it may be resumed; there is no need to start again.

b Reinforcing immunisation
A booster dose of vaccine containing diphtheria and tetanus toxoids is recommended for children immediately before school entry, preferably after at least three years from the last dose of the primary course.

6.3.2 Immunisation of persons aged ten years or over

a Primary immunisation
Diphtheria vaccine for adults (low dose) must be used because of the possibility of a serious reaction in an individual who is already immune. Three doses of 0.5ml should be given by deep subcutaneous or intramuscular injection at intervals of one month.

b Reinforcing immunisation

A single dose of 0.5ml is required. **This low-dose diphtheria vaccine must be used for all persons aged ten years and over; prior Schick testing is not necessary**.

6.3.3 Children given DTP at monthly intervals without a booster dose at 18 months have been shown to have adequate levels of diphtheria and tetanus antibody at school entry. A booster dose at 18 months for such children is therefore not necessary.

6.3.4 Contacts of a diphtheria case, or carriers of a toxigenic strain

Individuals exposed to such a risk should be given a complete course or a reinforcing dose according to their age and immunisation history as follows:

a   **Immunised** children up to ten years.
One injection of diphtheria vaccine.
b   **Immunised** children ten years and over, and adults.
One injection of diphtheria vaccine for adults (low dose).
c   **Unimmunised** children under ten years.
Three injections of diphtheria vaccine (or DTP and polio vaccines if appropriate) at monthly intervals.
d   **Unimmunised** children ten years and over, and adults.
Three injections of diphtheria vaccine for adults (low dose) at monthly intervals.

Unimmunised contacts of a case of diphtheria should in addition be given a prophylactic course of erythromycin.

6.3.5   HIV-positive individuals **may** be immunised against diphtheria in the absence of any contraindications (3.4).

6.4 Use of the Schick test

6.4.1   The Schick test is recommended for individuals who may be exposed to diphtheria in the course of their work. In such cases immunity to diphtheria should be ensured by means of a Schick test carried out at least three months after immunisation is completed.

6.5 Schick test

6.5.1   An intradermal injection of 0.2ml of Schick test toxin is given into the flexor surface of the left forearm and 0.2ml of Schick test control (inactivated toxin) material into the corresponding position of the right forearm, using separate syringes and needles. Readings should be made at 24-48 hours and five to seven days. Comparison of the appearances of the two injection sites will reveal responses attributable to immunity and to allergy. Four types of response may occur:

a   **Schick negative** – No visible reaction on either arm. The subject is **immune** and need not be immunised or reinforced.
b   **Schick positive** – An erythematous reaction develops at the site of the toxin injection, becoming evident in 24–48 hours and persisting for seven days or more before gradually fading. The control shows no reaction. The subject is **not immune** and requires to be immunised or reinforced.

c   **Negative-and-pseudo-reaction** – Both injection sites show similar reactions after 48–72 hours, which fade within five to six days. The reactions are due to hypersensitivity to the components of the test materials. The subject is IMMUNE and need NOT be immunised or reinforced.

d   **Positive-and-pseudo-reaction**
    Both injection sites show reactions after 48–72 hours but the reaction in the **left** arm (toxin) is usually larger and more intense than that on the **right** arm. The control response fades considerably by the fifth to seventh day leaving the positive effect clearly evident. Such combined reactors usually have a basal immunity to diphtheria and should **not** be immunised with a further full course of vaccine. Their immunity can successfully be reinforced by a single injection of diphtheria vaccine for adults (low-dose).

6.6   Adverse reactions

6.6.1   Swelling and redness at the injection site are common. Malaise, transient fever and headache may also occur. A small painless nodule may form at the injection site but usually disappears without sequelae. Severe anaphylactic reactions are rare. Neurological reactions have been reported occasionally.

6.6.2   Severe reactions should be reported to the Committee on Safety of Medicines using the yellow card system.

6.7   Contraindications

6.7.1

a   If a child is suffering from any acute illness, immunisation should be postponed until the child has fully recovered. Minor infections without fever or systemic upset are not reasons to postpone immunisation.

b   Immunisation should not proceed in children who have had a severe local or general reaction to a preceding dose, if it is thought that the diphtheria component has caused the preceding reaction. Reactions to the pertussis or tetanus components are more likely.

6.7.2   When there is a need to control an outbreak, diphtheria vaccine may have to be given to individuals suffering from acute febrile illness. **Low-dose diphtheria vaccine for adults must be used for persons aged ten years and over.**

6.8   Diphtheria antitoxin

6.8.1   Diphtheria antitoxin is now only used in suspected cases of diphtheria. Tests with a trial dose to exclude hypersensitivity should precede its use. It should be given without waiting for bacteriological confirmation since its action is specific for diphtheria. It may be given intramuscularly or intravenously, the dosage depending on the clinical condition of the patient. It is no longer used for diphtheria prophylaxis because of the risk of provoking a hypersensitivity reaction to the horse serum from which it is derived. Unimmunised contacts of a case of diphtheria should be promptly investigated, kept under surveillance and given antibiotic prophylaxis and vaccine as in 6.3.

6.9   Supplies

6.9.1   Diphtheria vaccines (6.2.2) **except** low-dose diphtheria vaccine for adults are manufactured and supplied by Evans Medical (Tel. 0403 41400). **Adsorbed vaccine must be specified or plain vaccine will be supplied**.

6.9.2   Low-dose diphtheria vaccine for adults is manufactured by Swiss Serum and Vaccine Institute, Berne, and distributed in the UK by Regent Laboratories Limited, Cunard Road, London NW10 6PN (Tel. 081-965 3637).

6.9.3   Schick Test Toxin and Schick Test Control BP. Manufactured and supplied by Evans Medical (Tel. 0403 41400).

6.9.4   Diphtheria antitoxin is supplied in vials containing 2000 Iu per ml. Manufactured by the Swiss Serum and Vaccine Institute, Berne, and distributed in the UK by Regent Laboratories Ltd. Cunard Road, London NW10 6PN (Tel. No. 081-965 3637).

6.10   Bibliography

Immunity of children to diphtheria, tetanus and poliomyelitis.
Bainton D, Freeman M, Magrath D, Sheffield F W, Smith J G W.
BMJ 1979; (1), 854-857.

Advantages of aluminium hydroxide adsorbed combined diphtheria, tetanus and pertussis vaccines for the immunisation of infants.
Butler N R, Voyce M A, Burland W M, Hilton M L.
BMJ 1959; (1), 663-666.

Susceptibility to diphtheria.
Report of Ad Hoc Working Group.
Lancet 1978; (i), 428-430.

Immunisation of adults against diphtheria.
Sheffield F W, Ironside A G, Abbott J D.
BMJ 1978; (2), 249-250.

Durability of immunity to diphtheria, tetanus and poliomyelitis after a three
dose immunisation schedule completed in the first eight months of life.
Jones E A, Johns A, Magrath D I, Melville-Smith M, Sheffield F.
Vaccine 1989: 7; 300-2.

7   Tetanus

7.1   Introduction

7.1.1   Tetanus is an acute disease characterised by muscular rigidity with superimposed agonising contractions. It is induced by the toxin of tetanus bacilli which grow anaerobically at the site of an injury. The incubation period is between four and 21 days, commonly about ten. Tetanus spores are present in soil and may be introduced into the body during injury, often through a puncture wound, but also through burns or trivial, unnoticed wounds. Neonatal tetanus due to infection of the baby's umbilical stump is an important cause of death in many countries in Asia and Africa, and cases still occur in the European region. World-wide elimination of neonatal tetanus by 1995 is one of the World Health Organisation targets. Tetanus is not spread from person to person.

7.1.2   Effective protection against tetanus is provided by active immunisation which was introduced in some localities as part of the primary immunisation of infants from the mid 1950's and nationally from 1961. Tetanus immunisation was provided by the Armed Forces from 1938. In 1970 it was recommended in the UK that active immunisation should be routinely provided in the treatment of wounds, when immunisation against tetanus should be initiated and subsequently completed.

7.1.3   Between 1985 and 1991 there were 104 cases of tetanus (notifications, deaths and laboratory reports) in England and Wales. 75% occurred in individuals over 45 years and of the reminder, 17% were in individuals from 25 to 44 years. 53% of all cases were in individuals over 65 years, two thirds of them being in women. Thus, the highest risk groups are the elderly with women being at greater risk than men.

Figures 7.1 and 7.2 show tetanus notifications for the period 1969 to 1991 and the distribution according to age and sex.

7.2   Tetanus vaccine and adsorbed tetanus vaccine

7.2.1   Immunisation protects by stimulating the production of antitoxin which provides immunity against the effects of the toxin. The immunogen is prepared by treating a cell-free preparation of toxin with formaldehyde and thereby converting it into the innocuous tetanus toxoid. This however is a relatively poor immunogen, and for use as a vaccine it is usually adsorbed onto an adjuvant, either aluminium phosphate or aluminium hydroxide. *Bordetella pertussis* also acts as an effective adjuvant.

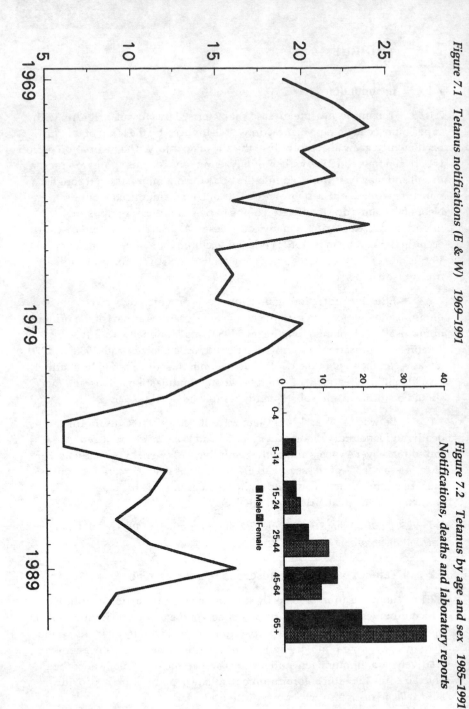

Figure 7.1 Tetanus notifications (E & W) 1969–1991

Figure 7.2 Tetanus by age and sex 1985–1991
Notifications, deaths and laboratory reports

The recommended vaccines for immunisation are:

> Adsorbed tetanus.
> Adsorbed diphtheria/tetanus.
> Adsorbed diphtheria/tetanus/pertussis.

Plain vaccines are less immunogenic and have no advantage in terms of reaction rates.

Vaccines should be stored at 2–8°C. The dose is 0.5ml given by intramuscular or deep subcutaneous injection.

7.3 Recommendations

7.3.1 For immunisation of infants and children under ten years.

a Primary immunisation

Triple vaccine, that is, vaccine containing diphtheria toxoid, tetanus toxoid, and *Bordetella pertussis*, is recommended for infants from two months of age. Adsorbed DTP vaccine should be used as it has been shown to cause fewer reactions than plain vaccine. If the pertussis component is contraindicated, adsorbed diphtheria/tetanus vaccine should be given. **A primary course of immunisation consists of three doses starting at two months with an interval of one month between each dose** (see 4.6). If a course is interrupted it may be resumed; there is no need to start again. The dose is 0.5ml given by intramuscular or deep subcutaneous injection.

b Reinforcing doses in children

A booster dose of adsorbed diphtheria/tetanus should be given prior to school entry, preferably with an interval of at least three years from the last dose of the primary course. If the primary course is only completed at school entry, then the booster dose should be given three years later. A further reinforcing dose of tetanus vaccine alone is recommended for those aged 15–19 years or before leaving school.

7.3.2 Children given DTP at monthly intervals without a booster dose of DT at 18 months have been shown to have adequate antibody levels at school entry. A booster dose at 18 months is therefore not recommended.

7.3.3 For immunisation of adults and children over ten years

Adults most likely to be susceptible to tetanus are the elderly, especially women, and men who have not served in the Armed Forces.

a For primary immunisation the course consists of three doses of 0.5ml of adsorbed tetanus vaccine by intramuscular or deep subcutaneous injection, with intervals of one month between each dose.

b A reinforcing dose ten years after the primary course and again ten years later maintains a satisfactory level of protection which will probably be life-long.

c For immunised adults who have received five doses, either in childhood, or as above, booster doses are not recommended, other than at the time of injury, since they have been shown to be unnecessary and can cause considerable local reactions.

7.3.4   Treatment of patients with tetanus-prone wounds

The following are considered tetanus-prone wounds:

a Any wound or burn sustained more than six hours before surgical treatment of the wound or burn.

b Any wound or burn at any interval after injury that shows one or more of the following characteristics:

(i) A significant degree of devitalised tissue.

(ii) Puncture-type wound.

(iii) Contact with soil or manure likely to harbour tetanus organisms.

(iv) Clinical evidence of sepsis.

Thorough surgical toilet of the wound is essential whatever the tetanus immunisation history of the patient.

Specific anti-tetanus prophylaxis

Immunisation Status	Type of Wound Clean	Type of Wound Tetanus Prone
Last of 3 dose course, or reinforcing dose within last 10 years	Nil	Nil – (A dose of adsorbed vaccine may be given if risk of infection is considered especially high, eg. contamination with stable manure).
Last of 3 dose course or reinforcing dose more than 10 years previously.	A reinforcing dose of adsorbed vaccine.	A reinforcing dose of adsorbed vaccine plus a dose of human tetanus immunoglobulin (7.3.5).
Not immunised or immunisation status not known with certainty.	A full 3 dose course adsorbed vaccine.	A full 3 dose course of vaccine, plus a dose of tetanus immunoglobulin in a different site.

7.3.5   Specific antitetanus immunoglobulin (see 4.10). See Table for recommendations.

Dose

Prevention: 250 Iu, or 500 Iu if more than 24 hours have elapsed since injury, or there is risk of heavy contamination or following burns.

Treatment: 150 Iu/kg given in multiple sites.

Available in 1ml ampoules containing 250 Iu.

7.3.6   Routine tetanus immunisation began in 1961, thus individuals born before that year will not have been immunised in infancy. After a tetanus-prone injury such individuals will therefore require a full course of immunisation unless it has previously been given, as for instance in the armed services.

7.3.7   Immunised individuals respond rapidly to a subsequent single injection of adsorbed tetanus vaccine, even after an interval of many years.

7.3.8   For wounds not in the above categories, such as clean cuts, antitetanus immunoglobulin should **not** be given.

7.3.9   Patients with impaired immunity who suffer a tetanus-prone wound may not respond to vaccine and may therefore require antitetanus immunoglobulin (7.3.5) in addition.

7.3.10   HIV-positive individuals **should** be immunised against tetanus in the absence of contraindications (7.5).

7.4   Adverse reactions

7.4.1   Local reactions, such as pain, redness and swelling round the injection site may occur and persist for several days. General reactions, which are uncommon, include headache, lethargy, malaise, myalgia and pyrexia. Acute anaphylactic reactions and urticaria may occasionally occur and, rarely, peripheral neuropathy. Persistent nodules at the injection site may arise if the injection is not given deeply enough.

7.4.2   Severe reactions should be reported to the Committee on Safety of Medicines using the yellow card system.

7.5   Contraindications

7.5.1

a   Tetanus vaccine should not be given to an individual suffering from acute febrile illness except in the presence of a tetanus-prone wound. Minor infections without fever or systemic upset are not reasons to postpone immunisation.

b   Immunisation should not proceed in individuals who have had a severe reaction to a previous dose (see 3.2.1 b.).

7.6   Supplies – vaccine

7.6.1   DTP and DT and T vaccines are manufactured by and available from Evans Medical (Tel. 0403 41400).

DT vaccine is also available from Merieux UK (Tel 0628 785291).

Adsorbed tetanus vaccine also available from:

Merieux UK (Tel. 0628 785291).
Servier Labs Ltd (Tel 0753 662744).

7.6.2   **Supplies – antitetanus immunoglobulin**

Bio Products Laboratory (Tel. 081 953 6191).
Regional Blood Transfusion Centres.
Evans (Humotet). (Tel 0403 41400).

Human tetanus immunoglobulin for intravenous use is available on a named patient basis from the Scottish National Blood Transfusion Service (Tel. 031 664 2317).

7.7   Bibliography

Prevention of tetanus in the wounded.
Smith J W G, Lawrence D R, Evans D G.
BMJ 1975: (iii) 453-455.

Immunity of children to diphtheria, tetanus and poliomyelitis.
Bainton D, Freeman M, Magrath D I, Sheffield F, Smith J W G.
BMJ 1979 (i) 854-857.

Excessive use of tetanus toxoid boosters.
Edsall G, Elliott M W, Peebles T C, Levine L, Eldred M C.
JAMA 1967 202 (i) 17-19.

Duration of immunity after active immunisation against tetanus.
White W G et al.
Lancet 1969 (ii) 95-96.

Reactions after plain and adsorbed tetanus vaccines.
White W G et al.
Lancet 1980 (i) 42.

To give or not to give; guidelines for tetanus vaccine.
Sheffield F W.
Community View (1985) 33, 8–9.

Durability of immunity to diphtheria, tetanus and poliomyelitis after a three dose schedule completed in the first eight months of life.
Jones E A, Johns A, Magrath D I, Melville-Smith M, Sheffield F.
Vaccine 1989: 7; 300-2.

8 Haemophilus influenzae type b (Hib)

8.1 Introduction

8.1.1 Infections due to *Haemophilus influenzae* are an important cause of morbidity and mortality, especially in young children. Invasive disease is usually caused by encapsulated strains of the organism. Six capsular serotypes (a-f) are known to cause disease in man; however, over 99% of typeable strains causing invasive disease are type b. Non-encapsulated strains are mainly associated with respiratory infections such as exacerbations of chronic bronchitis and otitis media.

8.1.2 The most common presentation of invasive Hib disease is meningitis, frequently accompanied by bacteraemia. This presentation accounts for approximately 60% of all cases. 15% of cases present with epiglottitis another potentially dangerous infection. Septicaemia, without any other concomitant infection, occurs in 10% of cases. The remainder is made up of cases of septic arthritis, osteomyelitis, cellulitis, pneumonia and pericarditis. The sequelae following Hib meningitis include deafness, convulsions and intellectual impairment. In studies conducted in Wales and Oxford, 8 to 11% had permanent neurological sequelae. The case fatality rate is 4 to 5%.

8.1.3 Based on the Wales and Oxford studies, the estimated annual incidence of invasive Hib disease is 34 per 100,000 children under the age of 5 years, ie. one in every 600 children develops disease before their fifth birthday. The number of laboratory reports in England and Wales increased from 869 in 1983 to 1259 in 1989.

8.1.4 The disease is rare in children under 3 months of age, but rises progressively during the first year, reaching a peak incidence between 10 and 11 months. Thereafter, the incidence declines steadily to 4 years of age after which infection becomes uncommon.

Figures 8.1 and 8.2 show the age distribution for reported Hib cases, October 1990 to December 1991.

8.1.5 Hib vaccine has been introduced into routine use in several countries. Finland, the first country to use the vaccine on a national scale, has shown a reduction from 203 cases in 1986 to only 12 cases in 1991.

8.2 Vaccine

8.2.1 Vaccines against Hib were first produced in the early 1970's. These vaccines contained purified capsular polysaccharide and were shown to be

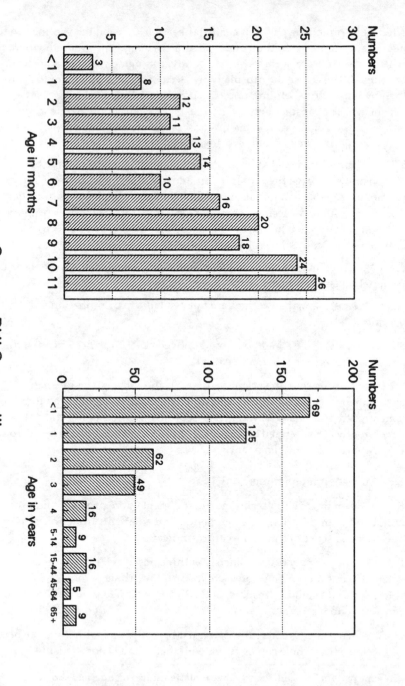

Figures 8.1 and 8.2   Age distribution of Hib cases   October 1990 to December 1991

Source: PHLS surveillance

effective in protecting children against disease. However, the vaccines were not immunogenic in children under 18 months of age, the group in whom the risks of disease were highest. More recently, conjugate vaccines have been developed. These take the capsular polysaccharides and link them to proteins, thereby improving their immunogenicity, especially in children less than one year of age. The capsular polysaccharides have been conjugated to diphtheria and tetanus toxoids, group B meningococcal outer membrane protein and a non-toxic derivative of diphtheria toxin.

8.2.2   The efficacy and safety of the conjugate Hib vaccines have been demonstrated in large field trials in Finland and the United States. Vaccine efficacy exceeds 95% in infants, immunised from 2 months of age. Studies comparing different vaccines, using the present United Kingdom primary schedule, have shown that 90 to 99% of children developed protective levels of antibody, following 3 doses.

8.2.3   The conjugate Hib vaccines are not live, containing non-replicating bacterial capsular antigens.

8.2.4   At present, the vaccines are not available in combination with other vaccines.

8.2.5   The vaccine should be stored between 2–8°C but not frozen. If the vaccine is frozen, it should not be used.

8.2.6   The dose of Hib vaccine is 0.5 ml. It should be given by deep subcutaneous or intramuscular injection, in a different limb from other concurrently administered vaccines. Recording the sites of injection of concurrently administered vaccines allows any local reactions to be attributed to the appropriate antigen or antigens.

8.3   Recommendations

8.3.1   Conjugate Hib vaccine, as a component of the primary course of childhood immunisation, is recommended for all infants from 2 months of age, in the absence of a genuine contra-indication.

8.3.2   The primary course consists of three doses of Hib vaccine with an interval of one month between each dose.[1] If the primary course is interrupted, it should be resumed allowing appropriate intervals between the remaining doses.

8.3.3   If a course is interrupted, it must be completed with **the same brand** of vaccine or the whole course repeated if that brand is not available.

---

[1] In some parts of Scotland, the schedule is started at two months and should be completed by six months, with intervals between injections of not less than one month.

8.3.4   No reinforcing (booster) doses are recommended for children who have received three injections at the appropriate times.

8.3.5   Children under the age of 13 months are at high risk of disease and should receive 3 doses of Hib vaccine, even if they have already commenced or completed their immunisations against Diphtheria, Tetanus, Pertussis and Poliomyelitis. Hib vaccine can be given at the same time as the other vaccines and any outstanding Hib doses should be given after the completion of the other antigens, separated by one month from the last Hib dose.

8.3.6   Children between 13 and 48 months should be given a single injection of Hib vaccine, either simultaneously with MMR vaccine, or singly if the MMR has already been given. Children in this age group are at lower risk of disease and the vaccine is effective after a single dose.

8.3.7   Because the incidence of invasive disease falls sharply after 4 years, routine immunisation of older children and adults is not recommended.

8.3.8   HIV positive individuals may receive Hib vaccine.

8.4   Adverse reactions

8.4.1   Swelling and redness at the injection site have been reported at a rate of up to 10%, following the first dose. However, the size of these reactions was rarely sufficient to contra-indicate further doses. These effects usually appear within 3 to 4 hours and resolve completely within 24 hours. The incidence of these reactions declines with subsequent doses, supporting the recommendation that courses of immunisation should be completed despite the occurrence of such reactions.

8.4.2   Following a severe local reaction, as defined at 3.2.1, further doses of Hib vaccine should not be given. Courses of DTP should be completed.

8.4.3   As Hib vaccine is given at the same time as DTP vaccine, it could be difficult to ascribe causality for a generalised reaction to any specific antigen. However, it has been shown that when Hib is given simultaneously with DTP, the incidence of generalised reactions is no greater than when DTP is given alone.

8.4.4   Despite more than 20 million doses of Hib vaccines having been administered to children, from 2 months of age, there have been no reports of serious adverse reactions attributed to the Hib vaccine.

8.5   Contraindications

8.5.1
a   If the child is suffering from any acute illness, immunisation should be

postponed until the child has recovered. Minor infections, without fever or systemic upset, are not reasons to postpone immunisation.

b   Immunisation should not proceed in children who have had a severe local reaction or a general reaction which can be confidently related to a preceding Hib immunisation. When Hib vaccine has been given with DTP, generalised reactions are far more likely to have been caused by the DTP vaccine.

8.6   Immunisation of contacts of Hib disease

8.6.1   Household contacts of a case of invasive Hib disease have an increased risk of contracting disease themselves. Any unimmunised household contact, under 4 years of age, should receive Hib vaccine (three doses if under 13 months, one dose if over 13 months and under 4 years). Independently of immunisation, rifampicin prophylaxis should be given.

8.6.2   The index case should also be immunised, irrespective of age.

8.6.3   When a case occurs in a playgroup, nursery or creche, the opportunity should be taken to identify and immunise any unimmunised children under 4 years of age. There is little evidence, however, that children in such settings are at significantly higher risk of Hib disease than the general population of the same age.

8.6.4   Hib vaccine is not a live vaccine, but there is no evidence at present of its safety in pregnancy.

8.7   Supplies

8.7.1   Because the currently available Hib vaccines are conjugated to markedly different proteins, it is unlikely that they are interchangeable. Thus, when a course is started with one vaccine, it must be completed with the same product. For this reason, only one product will be routinely available.

8.7.2   Hib vaccines are produced by:

> Merieux UK Tel 0628 785291
> Merck Sharpe & Dohme Tel 0992 467272
> Lederle Praxis (Cyanamid UK) Tel 0329 224000.

8.9   Bibliography

A survey of invasive Haemophilus influenzae infections
B Nazareth, M P E Slack, A J Howard, P A Waight, N T Begg
Communicable Disease Report
Vol 2: Review No 2: 31 January 1992

A randomised, prospective field trial of a conjugate vaccine in the protection of infants and young children against invasive Haemophilus influenzae type b disease
Eskola Juhani et al
New England Journal of Medicine
Vol 323: No. 20: 1991: 1381–1387

Immunisation of infants against Haemophilus influenzae type b in the UK
Booy R, Moxon E R
Archives of Disease in Childhood
1991: 66: 1251-1254

Efficacy in infancy of oligosaccharide conjugate Haemophilus influenzae type b (HbOC) vaccine in a United States population of 61 080 children
Black S B, Shinefield H R, Fireman B, Hiatt R, Polen M, Vittinghoff E
Pediatr Infect Dis J
1991: 10: 97-104

Safety and immunogenicity of oligosaccharide conjugate Haemophilus influenzae type b (HbOC) vaccine in infancy
Black S B, Shinefield H, Lampert D, Fireman B, Hiatt R A, Polen M, Vittinghoff E
Pediatr Infect Dis J
1991: Vol 10: No. 2

The efficacy in Navajo infants of a conjugate vaccine consisting of Haemophilus influenzae type b polysaccharide and neisseria meningitidis outer-membrane protein complex
Santosham M et al
The New England Journal of Medicine
Vol 324: No. 25: 1767

9 Poliomyelitis

9.1 Introduction

9.1.1 Poliomyelitis is an acute illness following invasion of the gastro-intestinal tract by one of the three types of polio virus (I, II and III). The virus has a high affinity for nervous tissue and the primary changes are in neurones. The infection may be clinically inapparent, or range in severity from a non-paralytic fever to aseptic meningitis or paralysis. Symptoms include headache, gastro-intestinal disturbance, malaise and stiffness of the neck and back, with or without paralysis. The infection rate in households with young children can reach 100%. The proportion of inapparent to paralytic infections may be as high as 1000 to one in children and 75 to one in adults, depending on the polio virus type and the social conditions. Poliomyelitis remains endemic in some developing countries where it occurs in epidemics. In countries where the disease incidence is low, but transmission is still occurring, polio cases are seen sporadically or as outbreaks amongst unimmunised individuals. Transmission is through contact with the faeces or pharyngeal secretions of an infected person.

9.1.2 The incubation period ranges from three to 21 days. Cases are most infectious from seven to ten days before and after the onset of symptoms; virus may be shed in the faeces for up to six weeks or longer.

9.1.3 Inactivated poliomyelitis vaccine (Salk) was introduced in 1956 for routine immunisation, and was replaced by attenuated live oral vaccine (Sabin) in 1962. **Individuals born before 1958 may not have been immunised and no opportunity should be missed to immunise them in adult life.** Since the introduction of vaccine, notifications of paralytic poliomyelitis (in E and W) have dropped from nearly 4,000 in 1955 to a total of 35 cases between 1974–1978. This included 25 cases during 1976 and 1977, in which infection with wild virus occurred in unimmunised persons, demonstrating the continuing need to maintain high levels of immunisation uptake. From 1985-91, 20 cases were reported. 13 were vaccine associated (9 recipients VA(R), 4 contacts VA(C)), 5 were imported; the source of infection could not be found in 3 cases, in none of whom could wild virus be detected.

Figure 9.1 shows poliomyelitis notifications from 1940 to 1991 and an analysis of polio reports, 1985 to 1992, by aetiology.

9.1.4 By May 1992, 92% of DHAs in England had achieved an uptake of 90% for poliomyelitis vaccine.

9.1.5 The World Health Organisation has included the UK among the

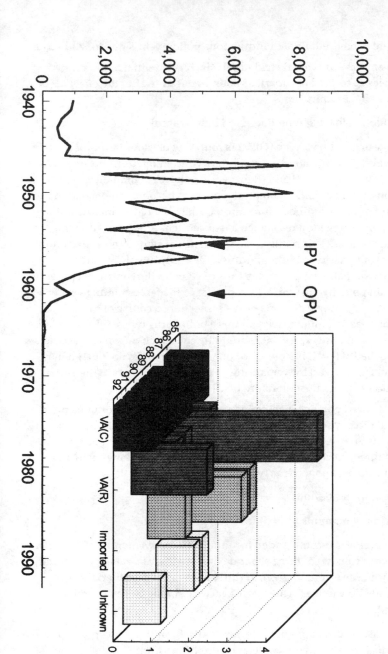

Figure 9.1 *Poliomyelitis notifications (E & W) 1940–1991 and by aetiology, 1985–1992*

countries which have eliminated indigenous poliomyelitis due to wild virus.

9.1.6   In any case of acute flaccid paralysis, it is essential to obtain two faecal samples 24 to 48 hours apart, as soon as possible after the onset of paralysis for viral examination.

9.2   Poliomyelitis vaccine (Live and Inactivated)

9.2.1   **Live oral polio vaccine (OPV)** is routinely used for immunisation in the UK, always given by mouth. It contains live attenuated strains of poliomyelitis virus types I, II and III grown in cultures of monkey kidney cells or on human diploid cells. The attenuated viruses become established in the intestine and promote antibody formation both in the blood and the gut epithelium, providing local resistance to subsequent infection with wild poliomyelitis viruses. This reduces the frequency of symptomless excretion of wild poliomyelitis virus in the community. OPV inhibits simultaneous infection by wild polio viruses and is thus of value in the control of epidemics. Vaccine strain poliomyelitis virus may persist in the faeces for up to six weeks after OPV. Whilst a single dose may give protection, a course of three doses produces long-lasting immunity to all three polio virus types. OPV should be stored at 0–4°C, and the expiry date should be checked before use. Vaccine stored unopened at 0–4°C is stable, but once the containers are open it may lose its potency. Any vaccine remaining in opened containers at the end of an immunisation session must therefore be discarded.

9.2.2   **Enhanced potency inactivated polio vaccine (eIPV)** contains polio viruses of all three types inactivated by formaldehyde. It should be stored at 0–4°C. 0.5ml is given by deep subcutaneous or intramuscular injection (9.3.9). A course of three injections at monthly intervals produces long-lasting immunity to all three polio virus types.

9.3   Recommendations

9.3.1   Primary immunisation of infants and children

Oral polio vaccine is recommended for infants from two months of age. **The primary course consists of three separate doses with intervals of one month between each dose (see 4.6), given at the same time as diphtheria/tetanus/ pertussis and Hib vaccines**. The dose of vaccine should be repeated if it is regurgitated.

9.3.2   Breast-feeding does not interfere with the antibody response to OPV and immunisation should not be delayed on this account.

9.3.3   Faecal excretion of vaccine virus which can last up to six weeks may lead to infection of unimmunised contacts; such infection may lead to protection of previously susceptible individuals, but see 3.4.5 and 9.3.9.

9.3.4   The contacts of a recently immunised baby should be advised of the need for strict personal hygiene, **particularly for washing their hands after changing the baby's napkins.**

Unimmunised adults can be immunised at the same time as their children (see 9.3.6). **There is no need to boost previously immunised individuals.**

9.3.5   Reinforcing immunisation in children

A reinforcing dose of oral poliomyelitis vaccine (OPV) should be given before school entry at the same time as the reinforcing dose of diphtheria and tetanus vaccine; a further dose of OPV should be given at 15–19 years of age or before leaving school.

9.3.6   **Immunisation of adults**

A course of three doses of OPV at intervals of four weeks is recommended for the primary immunisation of adults. **No adult should remain unimmunised against poliomyelitis (see 9.1.3).**

9.3.7   Reinforcing doses for adults are not necessary **unless** they are at special risk, such as:

a   Travellers to areas or countries where poliomyelitis is epidemic or endemic. (See "Health advice for travellers" T4 1992.)

b   Health care workers in possible contact with poliomyelitis cases.

9.3.8   For those exposed to a continuing risk of infection a single reinforcing dose is desirable every ten years.

9.3.9   Inactivated polio vaccine (IPV) is available for the immunisation of individuals for whom a live vaccine is contra-indicated (see 3.2.1 (iv)). It should also be used for siblings and other household contacts of immuno-suppressed individuals. A primary course of three doses of 0.5ml with intervals of one month should be given by deep subcutaneous or intramuscular injection. Reinforcing doses should be given as for OPV.

9.3.10   HIV-positive asymptomatic individuals **may** receive live polio vaccine but excretion of the vaccine virus in the faeces may continue for longer than in normal individuals. Household contacts should be warned of this and for the need for strict personal hygiene, including hand-washing after nappy changes for an HIV-positive infant.

9.3.11   For HIV-positive symptomatic individuals, IPV may be used instead of OPV at the discretion of the clinician.

Poliomyelitis

9.4   Adverse reactions

9.4.1   Cases of vaccine-associated poliomyelitis have been reported in recipients of OPV and in contacts of recipients. In England and Wales there is an annual average of one recipient and one contact case in relation to over two million doses of oral vaccine. Contact cases would be eliminated if all children and adults were immunised. The possibility of a very small risk of poliomyelitis induced by OPV cannot be ignored but is insufficient to warrant a change in immunisation policy. **The need for strict personal hygiene for contacts of recent vaccinees must be stressed.**

9.4.2   Such cases following immunisation with poliomyelitis vaccine (9.4.1) should be reported to the Committee on Safety of Medicines using the yellow card system.

9.5   Contraindications

(i)   Acute or febrile illness; immunisation should be postponed.

(ii)   Vomiting or diarrhoea; immunisation should be postponed.

(iii)   Treatment involving high-dose corticosteroids or immuno-suppression including general radiation (see 3.2.1 (iii) & (iv)).

(iv)   Malignant conditions of the reticulo-endothelial system such as lymphoma, leukaemia, and Hodgkin's disease, and where the normal immunological mechanism may be impaired as for example, in hypogammaglobulinaemia. See also 3.2.1 (iii) & (iv).

(v)   Although adverse effects on the fetus have not been reported, oral polio vaccine should not be given to women during the first four months of pregnancy unless there are compelling reasons, such as travel to an endemic poliomyelitis area.

9.5.1   OPV **may** be given at the same time as inactivated vaccines and with other live virus vaccines except oral typhoid vaccine (see 20.9.1.d). If not given simultaneously with other live virus vaccines, an interval of three weeks should be observed. However, when BCG if given to infants, there is no need to delay the primary immunisations which include polio vaccine, because the latter viruses replicate in the intestine to induce local immunity and serum antibodies, and three doses are given.

9.5.2   Both OPV and IPV may contain trace amounts of penicillin and streptomycin but these do not contraindicate their use except in cases of extreme hypersensitivity. Both vaccines contain neomycin in small amounts and OPV may also contain polymyxin.

9.5.3   OPV should **not** be used for the siblings and other household contacts of immunosuppressed children; such contacts should be given IPV.

9.5.4   OPV should be given either three weeks before or three months after an injection of normal immunoglobulin – for instance for hepatitis A (see Section 15). This may not always be possible in the case of travellers going abroad, but as in such cases the OPV is likely to be a booster dose the possible inhibiting effect of immunoglobulin is less important.

9.6   Management of outbreaks

9.6.1   After a single case of paralytic poliomyelitis from wild virus, a dose of OPV should be given to all persons in the immediate neighbourhood of the case (with the exception of individuals with genuine contraindications such as immunodeficiency, to whom IPV should be given, see 9.3.9), regardless of a previous history of immunisation against poliomyelitis. **In previously unimmunised individuals the three dose course must be completed**. If there is laboratory confirmation that a vaccine-derived polio virus is responsible for the case, immunisation of further possible contacts is unnecessary since no outbreaks associated with vaccine virus have been documented to date. If the source of the outbreak is uncertain, it should be assumed to be a "wild" virus and appropriate control measures instituted.

9.7   Supplies

9.7.1

a   Oral poliomyelitis vaccine is available in 10 x 1 dose packs and in dropper tubes of ten doses from:

Evans Medical (Tel. 0403 41400).
SmithKline Beecham Ltd. (0707 325111).

b   Inactivated polio vaccine (IPV) is supplied in single dose 1ml ampoules. Obtained from:

Department of Health, 14 Russell Square, WC18 5EP
Tel. 071-636 6811.

Welsh Health Common Service Authority, Cardiff. Tel. 0222 471234.

Central Services Agency, 25 Adelaide Street, Belfast BT2 8FH Tel. 0232 324431

9.8   Bibliography

Paralytic poliomyelitis in England and Wales 1976–77.
Collingham K E, Pollock T M, Roebuck M O.
Lancet 1978: (i); 976-977.

Effect of breast feeding on sero-response of infants to oral polio vaccine.
John T J, et al.
Pediatrics 1976: 57; 47-53.

Paralytic poliomyelitis in England and Wales 1970-84.
Begg N T, Chamberlain R, Roebuck M.
Epidem Inf 1987: 99; 97-106.

Immunity of children to diphtheria, tetanus and poliomyelitis.
Bainton D, Freeman M, Magrath D I et al.
BMJ 1979: (i); 854-857.

Prevalence of antibodies to polio virus in 1978 among subjects aged 0–88 years.
Roebuck M, Chamberlain R.
BMJ 1982: 284; 697-700.

Prevalence of antibody to polio virus in England and Wales 1984–86.
White P, Green J.
BMJ 1986: 293; 1153-1155.

10 Measles, Mumps, Rubella –

(for Rubella see also Section 11)

10.1 Introduction

10.1.1   In 1988 combined measles/mumps/rubella (MMR) vaccine was introduced in the UK for young children of both sexes with the aim of eliminating measles, mumps, rubella and the Congenital Rubella Syndrome (CRS). MMR vaccine replaces single antigen measles vaccine; by giving the rubella component to young children it is intended to interrupt the circulation of rubella and thereby remove the risk of infection to non-immune pregnant women. **Rubella immunisation of girls and non-immune women continues (Section 11)**.

10.1.2 **Measles** is an acute viral illness transmitted via droplet infection. Clinical features include Koplik spots, coryza, conjunctivitis, bronchitis, rash and fever. The incubation period is about ten days, with a further two to four days before the rash appears. It is highly infectious from the beginning of the prodromal period to four days after the appearance of the rash. Complications have been reported in one in 15 notified cases, and include otitis media, bronchitis, pneumonia, convulsions, and encephalitis, which has an incidence of one in 5000 cases, has a mortality of about 15%, and 20 to 40% of survivors have residual neurological sequelae. Electro-encephalographic changes have been reported after apparently uncomplicated measles as well as in cases with frank encephalitis. Complications are more common and severe in poorly nourished and chronically ill children; **it is therefore particularly important that such children should be immunised against measles**.

10.1.3   Notification of measles began in England and Wales in 1940, and until the introduction of vaccine in 1968 annual notifications varied between 160,000 and 800,000, the peaks occurring in two year cycles. By the mid-seventies notifications had fallen to between 50,000 and 180,000. Deaths from measles declined from 1000 in 1940 to 90 in 1968; after the introduction of immunisation the decline continued to an annual average of 13 deaths in the period 1970 to 1988. More than half the deaths occurred in previously healthy unimmunised children. Measles was a major cause of morbidity and mortality in children receiving immunosuppressive treatment, particularly for leukaemia. Between 1970 and 1983, 19 children in remission from acute lymphatic leukaemia died from measles, and of 51 children who died in their first remission in 1974-84, measles was the cause in nearly a third. An additional average of ten deaths a year result from subacute sclerosing panencephalitis, a rare but fatal late complication of measles infection.

10.1.4   Since the introduction of MMR vaccine in October 1988, notifications of measles have fallen progressively to the lowest levels since records began in 1940. In 1991, there were only 9985 measles notifications. Recent research suggests that many of the notified cases of sporadic measles are not confirmed by laboratory tests [PHLS unpublished data]. **In 1990 and 1991, no single child died of acute measles related illness in England and Wales.**

Figure 10.1 shows notifications of measles from 1940 to 1991.

10.1.5   From 1968 to 1980 measles vaccine uptake for children aged one to two years remained between 50% and 60%. However by May 1992, the overall figure had increased to 92%, with 77% of Health Authorities in England, Wales and Northern Ireland, achieving an uptake of over 90%.

10.1.6   **Mumps** is an acute viral illness characterised by parotid swelling which may be unilateral or bilateral; some cases are asymptomatic. The incubation period is 14–21 days and mumps is transmissible from several days before the parotid swelling to several days after it appears. Complications include pancreatitis, oophoritis and orchitis; even when the latter is bilateral there is no firm evidence that it causes sterility. Neurological complications including meningitis and encephalitis may precede or follow parotitis, and can also occur in its absence. Before the introduction of MMR vaccine, mumps was the cause of about 1200 hospital admissions each year in England and Wales. In the under 15 age group it was a common cause of viral meningitis; it can also cause permanent unilateral deafness at any age.

10.1.7   Mumps was made a notifiable disease in the UK in October 1988.

10.1.8   Notifications have fallen progressively; in 1991 there were 2924 notifications. If current levels of uptake of vaccine are maintained, then interruption of transmission can be expected, leading to mumps elimination.

Figure 10.2 shows the rates of mumps reports to the Royal College of General Practitioners from 1985 to 1992.

10.1.9   **Rubella** is a mild infectious disease, most common among children aged four to nine years. It causes a transient erythematous rash, lymphadenopathy involving post-auricular and sub-occipital glands and occasionally in adults, arthritis and arthralgia. Clinical diagnosis is unreliable since the symptoms are often fleeting and can be caused by other viruses; in particular, the rash is not diagnostic of rubella. **A history of "rubella" should never be accepted without serological evidence of previous infection (11.1.4).** The incubation period is 14–21 days and the period of infectivity from one week before until four days after the onset of rash.

10.1.10   Maternal rubella infection in the first eight to ten weeks of pregnancy

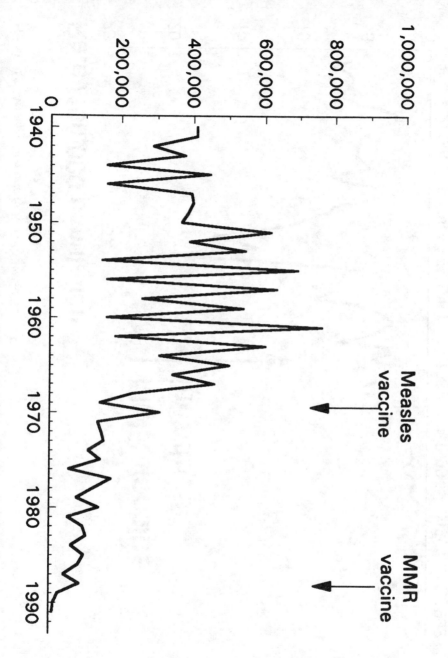

Figure 10.1   Measles notifications (E & W)   1940–1991

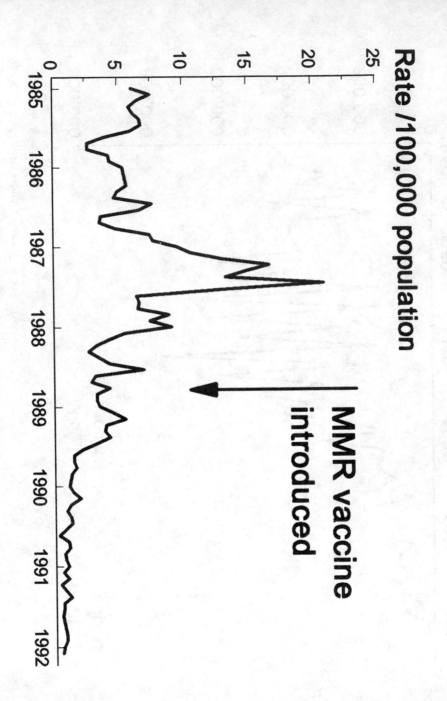

Figure 10.2 Mumps Reports to RCGP 1985–1992

Rate /100,000 population

MMR vaccine introduced

Measles/Mumps/Rubella (MMR)

results in fetal damage in up to 90% of infants and multiple defects are common. The risk of damage declines to about 10–20% by 16 weeks and after this stage of pregnancy, fetal damage is rare. Fetal defects include mental handicap, cataract, deafness, cardiac abnormalities, retardation of intra-uterine growth and inflammatory lesions of brain, liver, lungs and bone-marrow. Any combination of these may occur; the only defects which commonly occur alone are perceptive deafness and pigmentary retinopathy following infection after the first eight weeks of pregnancy. Some infected infants may appear normal at birth but perceptive deafness may be detected later. **For investigation of suspected rubella or exposure to rubella in pregnant women see Section 11**.

10.1.11   Rubella immunisation was introduced in the UK in 1970 for pre-pubertal girls and non-immune women with the aim of protecting women of child-bearing age from the risks of rubella in pregnancy. This policy was not intended to prevent the circulation of rubella, but to increase the proportion of women with antibody to rubella; this increased from 85-90% before 1970 to 97–98% by 1987.

10.1.12   Rubella was made a notifiable disease in the UK in 1988, since which time, notifications have progressively fallen. For reporting of CRS see Section 11.8.

10.2   MMR Vaccine

10.2.1   This is a freeze-dried preparation containing live attenuated measles, mumps and rubella viruses. It must be stored in the dry state at 2–8°C (**not** frozen) and protected from light. It should be reconstituted with the diluent supplied by the manufacturer and used within one hour. A single dose of 0.5ml is given by intramuscular or deep subcutaneous injection. Immunisation results in sero-conversion to all three viruses in over 95% of recipients; vaccine-induced antibody to rubella has been shown to persist for at least 16 years in the absence of endemic disease. Since the vaccine viruses are not transmitted, there is **no risk of infection** from vaccinees.

Three vaccines are currently available:

Pluserix-MMR (SmithKline Beecham); Schwartz strain measles, RA 27/3 rubella, Urabe Am/9 mumps.

MMR II (Wellcome); Enders' Edmonston strain measles, RA 27/3 rubella, Jeryl Lynn mumps.

Immravax (Merieux UK); Schwartz strain measles, RA 27/3 rubella Urabe Am/9 mumps.

10.2.2   Single antigen measles, mumps and rubella vaccines are still available. (See Section 11 for Rubella).

10.2.3   **Single antigen rubella vaccine will continue to be given to girls aged 10–14 years if they have not previously received MMR vaccine, and to non-immune women before pregnancy and after delivery: see Section 9.**

10.3   Recommendations

10.3.1   MMR vaccine is recommended for children of both sexes aged 12 to 15 months unless there is a genuine contraindication (see 10.5). It is also recommended for pre-school children who have not previously received it. **MMR vaccine should be given irrespective of a history of measles, mumps or rubella infection or measles immunisation. There are no ill effects from immunising such children**.

10.3.2   MMR vaccine can be given to children **of any age** whose parents request it, and no opportunity should be missed to ensure that this is done. If the primary immunisations have not been completed at the time that MMR vaccine is due, they can be given at the same time using separate syringes and different sites. Similarly, if children who attend for pre-school immunisation (D/T/polio) have not received MMR vaccine, it should be given then. However since measles, mumps and rubella are most common before the age of entry to secondary school, mass immunisation after the age of 11 when 80–90% have already acquired antibody would currently have little effect on the disease incidence. For maximum effect, vaccine must be given soon after the first birthday, and at the latest before the age of five.

10.3.3   In areas where uptake was low in the past, there may be cohorts of increasing age who are still susceptible to measles. Such groups may provide foci for measles outbreaks especially in schools. Where older unimmunised children can be identified, they should be immunised with MMR vaccine.

10.3.4   If parents do not wish DT and MMR vaccine to be given at the same visit, then OPV should be given with MMR and the child recalled for the DT booster as soon as possible; in these circumstances no three week interval between immunisations is necessary.

10.3.5   MMR vaccine can be given to non-immune adults and should be considered for those in long-term institutional care who may not have developed immunity.

10.3.6   Children with a personal or close family history of convulsions **should** be given MMR vaccine, provided the parents understand that there may be a febrile response. As for all children, advice for reducing fever should be given (10.4.4). Doctors should seek specialist paediatric advice rather than refuse immunisation. Dilute immunoglobulin as formerly used with measles vaccine for such children is no longer used since it may inhibit the immune response to the rubella and mumps components.

10.3.7 Unimmunised children in the following groups are at particular risk from measles infection and **should** be immunised with MMR vaccine:

a Children with chronic conditions such as cystic fibrosis, congenital heart or kidney disease, failure to thrive, Down's syndrome.
b Children from the age of one year upwards in residential or day care, including playgroups and nursery schools.

10.3.8 As vaccine-induced **measles** antibody develops more rapidly than that following natural infection, MMR vaccine can be used to protect susceptible contacts during a **measles** outbreak. To be effective the vaccine must be administered within three days of exposure. If there is doubt about a child's immunity, vaccine should be given since there are no ill effects from immunising individuals who are already immune. Immunoglobulin is available for individuals for whom vaccine is contraindicated (10.5).

NB. **Antibody responses to the rubella and mumps components of MMR vaccine are too slow for effective prophylaxis after exposure to these infections.**

10.3.9 Reimmunisation is only necessary when vaccine has been given before 12 months of age.

10.3.10 Measles virus inhibits the response to tuberculin, so tuberculin-positive individuals may become tuberculin-negative for up to a month after measles infection or MMR vaccine. Because the measles virus may cause exacerbation of tuberculosis, such patients should be under treatment when immunised.

10.3.11 HIV-positive individuals **may** be given MMR vaccine in the absence of contraindications (10.5).

10.4 Adverse reactions

10.4.1 Malaise, fever and/or a rash may occur, most commonly about a week after immunisation and last about two to three days. In a study of over 6000 children aged one to two years, the symptoms reported were similar in nature, frequency, time of onset and duration to those commonly reported after measles vaccine. During the sixth to eleventh days after vaccine, febrile convulsions occurred in 1/1000 children, the rate previously reported in the same period after measles vaccine. Parotid swelling occurred in about 1% of children of all ages up to four years, usually in the third week and occasionally later.

10.4.2   Culture positive mumps meningo-encephalitis occurs at a rate of approximately one case per 300,000 distributed doses of vaccine using the Urabe mumps virus containing vaccines but higher rates have been reported from some localities. The rate following Jeryl Lynn mumps vaccine is lower. All cases reported between 1988 and 1992 are being carefully followed up. When mumps virus is isolated from the cerebro-spinal fluid in such cases, laboratory tests can distinguish between wild and vaccine strains. Advice should be sought from the National Institute for Biological Standards and Control (Tel. 0707 54753).

10.4.3   Thrombocytopenia, which is usually self-limiting, is occasionally associated with the rubella component.

10.4.4   Parents should be told about possible symptoms and given advice for reducing fever, including the use of paracetamol in the period five to ten days after immunisation. They should also be reassured that post-immunisation symptoms are **not** infectious.

10.4.5   Serious reactions should be reported to the Committee on Safety of Medicines using the yellow card system.

10.5   Contraindications

(i)   Children with acute febrile illness when they present for immunisation; this should be deferred.

(ii)   Children with untreated malignant disease or altered immunity; those receiving immunosuppressive or X-ray therapy or high-dose steroids (3.2.1 (iii), (iv) & (v) and 10.7).

(iii)   Children who have received another live vaccine – including BCG – within three weeks.

(iv)   Children with allergies to neomycin or kanamycin.

(v)   If MMR vaccine is given to adult women, pregnancy should be avoided for one month, as for rubella vaccine (11.3.2 and 11.5.1).

(vi)   MMR vaccine should not be given within three months of an injection of immunoglobulin.

10.5.1   Allergy to egg

This is only a contraindication if the child has had an anaphylactic reaction (generalised urticaria, swelling of the mouth and throat, difficulty in breathing, hypotension or shock) following food containing egg. Dislike of egg or refusal to eat it is **not** a contraindication. If there is genuine concern, paediatric advice should be sought with a view to immunisation under controlled conditions such as hospital day case admission.

10.6   Supplies

Pluserix-MMR. SmithKline Beecham Tel. 0707 325111.
MMR II. Merck, Sharp and Dohme Tel. 0992 467272
Immravax. Merieux UK Tel. 0628 785291.

10.7   Immunoglobulin

10.7.1   Measles

Children and adults with compromised immunity (3.2.1 iii, iv, & v) who come into contact with measles should be given human normal immunoglobulin (HNIG) as soon as possible after exposure. Testing for measles antibody may delay the administration of HNIG and neither immunisation nor low level antibody guarantees immunity to measles in the immuno compromised.

Children under 12 months in whom there is a particular reason to avoid measles, (such as recent severe illness), can also be given immunoglobulin; MMR vaccine should then be given after an interval of at least three months, at around the usual age.

Dose:

	Age	Dose
To prevent an attack:		
	Under 1 year	250 mg
	1–2 years	500 mg
	3 and over	750 mg
To allow an attenuated attack:		
	Under 1 year	100 mg
	1 year or over	250 mg

An interval of at least three months must be allowed before subsequent MMR immunisation.

Dilute immunoglobulin as previously used with measles vaccine for children with a history of convulsions is no longer used since it may inhibit the immune response to rubella and mumps.

10.7.2 Mumps

HNIG is no longer used for post-exposure protection since there is no evidence that it is effective. Mumps-specific immunoglobulin is no longer available.

10.7.3 Rubella

Post-exposure prophylaxis does **not** prevent infection in non-immune contacts and is therefore **not** recommended for the protection of pregnant women exposed to rubella. It may however reduce the likelihood of clinical symptoms which may possibly reduce the risk to the fetus. It should only be used when termination of pregnancy for proved rubella infection is unacceptable, when it should be given as soon as possible after exposure; serological follow-up of recipients is essential.

Dose: 750 mg

10.7.4 Supplies of HNIG:

Central Public Health Laboratory. Tel. 081 200 6868
Public Health Laboratories, England and Wales
Blood Transfusion Service, Scotland
Bio Products Laboratory Tel. 081 953 6191.
The Laboratories, Belfast City Hospital Tel. 0232 329241.
Immuno, Tel. 0732 458101. (Gammabulin).
Kabivitrum, Tel. 0895 51144 (Kabiglobulin).

10.8 Bibliography

Severity of notified measles.
Miller C L.
BMJ 1978; i: 1253.

Deaths from measles.
Miller C L.
BMJ 1985; 290: 443-444.

Mortality and morbidity caused by measles in children with malignant disease attending four major treatment centres: a retrospective view.
Gray M, Hann I M, Glass S, Eden O B, Morris Jones P, Stevens R F.
BMJ 1987; 295: 19–22.

Measles serology in children with a history of measles in early life.
Adjaye N, Azad A, Foster M, Marshall W C, Dunn H.
BMJ 1983; 286: 1478.

Live measles vaccine: a 21 year follow up.
Miller C L.
BMJ 1987; 295: 22-24.

Safe administration of mumps/measles/rubella vaccine in egg-allergic children.
Greenberg M A, Birx D L.
J. Pediatrics 1988; 113: 504-6.

Safe immunisation of allergic children against measles, mumps and rubella.
Juntenen-Backman K, Peltola H, Backman A, Salo O P.
Am. J. Dis. Children 1987; 141: 1103–5.

Virus meningitis and encephalitis in 1979.
Noah N D, Urquart A M.
J. Infection 1980; 2: 379–83.

Big bang for immunisation. Editorial.
Sir John Badenoch.
BMJ 1988; 297: 750–1.

Surveillance of antibody to measles, mumps and rubella by age.
Morgan-Capner P, Wright J, Miller C L, Miller E.
BMJ 1988; 297: 770–2.

Surveillance of symptoms following MMR vaccine in children.
Miller C L et al.
Practitioner 1989; 233: 69-73.

Mumps meningitis and MMR vaccination.
Lancet 1989, ii: 1015-1016.

Mumps viruses and mumps, measles, and rubella vaccine.
Forsey T, Minor P D.
BMJ 1989; 299: 1340.

Egg hypersensitivity and measles/mumps/rubella vaccine administration.
Beck SA, Williams L W, Shirrell M, Burks A W
Paediatrics 1991; 88: 5: 913-917.

Vaccine safety versus vaccine efficacy in mass immunisation programmes
Nokes D J Anderson R M
Lancet 1991: 338: 1309-1312

For rubella references see Section 11.

11   Rubella

11.1   Introduction

11.1.1   Rubella is a mild infectious disease, most common among children aged four to nine years. It causes a transient erythematous rash, lymphadenopathy involving post-auricular and sub-occipital glands and occasionally in adults, arthritis and arthralgia. Clinical diagnosis is unreliable since the symptoms are often fleeting and can be caused by other viruses; in particular the rash is not diagnostic of rubella. **A history of rubella should therefore not be accepted without serological evidence of previous infection**. The incubation period is 14–21 days, and the period of infectivity is from one week before until four days after the onset of rash

11.1.2   Maternal rubella infection in the first eight to ten weeks of pregnancy results in fetal damage in up to 90% of infants and multiple defects are common, the Congenital Rubella Syndrome (CRS). The risk of damage declines to about 10-20% by 16 weeks; after this stage of pregnancy fetal damage is rare. Fetal defects include mental handicap, cataract, deafness, cardiac abnormalities, retardation of intra-uterine growth, and inflammatory lesions of brain, liver, lungs and bone-marrow. Any combination of these defects may occur; the only defects which commonly occur alone are perceptive deafness and pigmentary retinopathy following infection after the first eight weeks of pregnancy. Some infected infants may appear normal at birth but perceptive deafness may be detected later. In 1991, there were only 15 laboratory confirmed rubella infections in pregnant women, reported to CDSC, compared with 164 in 1987. Rubella associated terminations of pregnancy fell from 738 in 1972 to 10 in 1990. Since the introduction of MMR vaccine, CRS cases, reported to the National Congenital Rubella Surveillance Programme, have fallen to around 10 cases annually.

Figure 11.1 shows reports of laboratory confirmed rubella in pregnant women and children less than 15 years, 1975 to 1991.

11.1.3   Rubella was made a notifiable disease in the UK in 1988. For notification of cases of CRS see 11.8.

11.1.4   Confirmation of rubella infection in pregnant women

Because the rash is not diagnostic and also because infection can occur with no clinical symptoms, acute rubella can only be confirmed by laboratory tests.

11.1.5   Investigation of pregnant women exposed to rubella

All pregnant women with suspected rubella or exposed to rubella must be

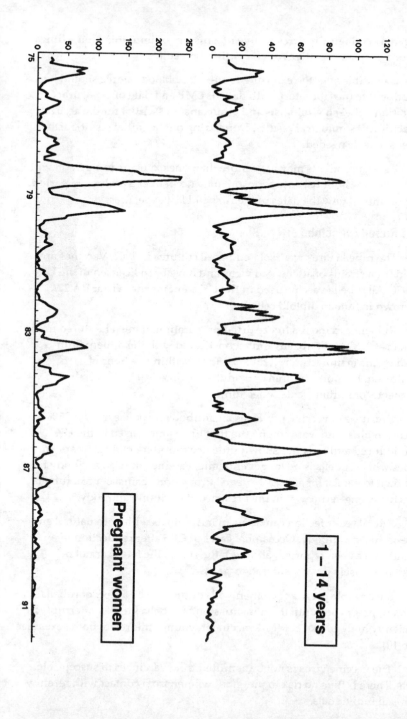

Figure 11.1 Reports of laboratory confirmed rubella in pregnant women and children <15y
Source PHLS

1 – 14 years

Pregnant women

investigated serologically, irrespective of a history of immunisation, clinical rubella or a previous positive rubella antibody result.

As soon as possible after the exposure to rubella, a blood sample should be taken and sent to the laboratory with **date of LMP and date of exposure. Close collaboration between virologists and clinicians is essential for the accurate interpretation of serological results.** Depending on the initial result, further specimens may be needed.

11.1.6   As some patients may have more than one exposure to a person with a rubella like illness, or because exposure may occur over a prolonged period, it is important to know the dates of the first and last exposures.

11.2   Rubella vaccine

11.2.1   The rubella virus was isolated in cell cultures in 1962. Vaccines are prepared from strains of attenuated virus and have been licensed in the UK since 1970. All rubella vaccine used in the UK contains the Wistar RA 27/3 strain grown in human diploid cells.

11.2.2   Rubella vaccine is a freeze dried preparation. It must be stored in the dried state at 2–8°C (**not** frozen) and reconstituted with the diluent fluid supplied by the manufacturer; it must be used within one hour of reconstitution. For both children and adults the dose is 0.5ml given by subcutaneous or intramuscular injection.

11.2.3   One dose of vaccine produces an antibody response in over 95% of vaccinees. In girls who were among the first to be immunised in the UK, vaccine-induced antibody has shown little decline after nearly 20 years. In countries where rubella is no longer endemic, vaccine-induced antibody has been shown to persist for at least 16 years. Protection against clinical rubella appears to be long-term even in the presence of declining antibody.

11.2.4   Rubella re-infection can occur in individuals with both natural and vaccine-induced antibody. Occasional cases of CRS after reinfection in pregnancy have been reported; although the risk to the fetus cannot be quantified precisely it is considered to be low.

11.2.5   Susceptible pregnant women will continue to be at risk of rubella infection in pregnancy until the transmission of rubella virus is interrupted by a sufficiently high uptake of MMR vaccine in young children of both sexes (see Section 10).

11.2.6   The vaccine virus is not transmitted from vaccinees to susceptible contacts. There is thus no risk to pregnant women from contact with recently immunised individuals.

11.3   Recommendations

11.3.1

a   All girls between their 10th and 14th birthdays should be immunised with single antigen rubella vaccine unless there is documented evidence that they have received MMR vaccine already. A history of rubella should be disregarded because of the unreliability of diagnosis. Serological testing of these girls before immunisation need not be undertaken, nor enquiry into LMP, given the rarity of pregnancy in this age group, the likely irregularity of menstruation and the very low risk of immunisation in pregnancy having any adverse effect (see 11.3.2).

Single antigen rubella vaccine will continue to be given to girls aged 10–14 years if they have not previously received MMR vaccine, and to non-immune women before pregnancy and after delivery.

This programme will continue with the present target of 95% in order to maintain the current high proportion of women with rubella antibody.

b   Non-pregnant seronegative women of child-bearing age should be given single antigen rubella vaccine and advised not to become pregnant within one month of immunisation.

Female immigrants who have entered the UK after the age of school immunisation are particularly likely to require immunisation. Approximately one in five of the children currently born with congenital rubella syndrome is of Asian origin.

11.3.2   Immunisation should be avoided in early pregnancy; doctors should ascertain the date of the LMP before immunising. However despite active surveillance in USA, UK and Germany no case of Congenital Rubella Syndrome has been reported following inadvertent immunisation shortly before or during pregnancy (but see 11.8.1 and 11.8.2). There is thus no evidence that the vaccine is teratogenic; termination of pregnancy following immunisation should therefore **not** be recommended. The potential parents should be given this information before considering termination.

11.3.3.   General practitioners are uniquely placed to ensure that all women of child-bearing age have been screened for rubella antibody and immunised where necessary. Opportunities for screening also arise during ante-natal care, and at family planning, infertility and occupational health clinics. In such cases general practitioners must be informed of the results. Every effort must be made to identify and immunise sero-negative women. **All women should be informed of the result of their antibody test.**

11.3.4   Women should be screened for rubella antibodies in every pregnancy, and on request when pregnancy is contemplated, irrespective of a previous positive rubella antibody result. One quarter of the small number of women currently being infected during pregnancy had been reported to be immune in the past. Very occasionally, laboratory errors or errors during reporting may result in patients who are sero-negative being reported as sero-positive.

11.3.5   Serological testing of non-pregnant women should be performed whenever possible before immunisation but need not be undertaken where this might interfere with the acceptance or delivery of vaccine. Pregnancy should be avoided for one month.

11.3.6   Women found to be seronegative on ante-natal screening should be immunised after delivery and before discharge from the maternity unit. If anti-D immunoglobulin is required, the two may be given at the same time in different sites with separate syringes. While it has now been established that anti-D immunoglobulin does not interfere with the antibody response to vaccine, blood transfusion does inhibit the response in up to 50% of vaccinees. In such cases a test for antibody should be performed eight weeks later, with reimmunisation if necessary. If rubella vaccine is not given post-partum before discharge, the general practitioner **must** be informed of the need for this. Alternatively it can be given at the post-natal visit. The risk of rubella infection in pregnancy has been greater for parous than for nulliparous women because their own children were a source of infection. **All women found on antenatal screening to be susceptible to rubella should be immunised after delivery and before the next pregnancy**.

11.3.7   To avoid the risk of transmitting rubella to pregnant patients, **all health service staff, both male and female**, should be screened and those seronegative immunised.

11.3.8   Rubella vaccine **may** be given to HIV positive individuals in the absence of contraindications (11.5).

11.4   Adverse reactions

11.4.1   Mild reactions such as fever, sore throat, lymphadenopathy, rash, arthralgia and arthritis may occur following immunisation. Symptoms usually begin one to three weeks after immunisation and are transient; joint symptoms are more common in women than in young girls. Thrombocytopenia, usually self-limiting, has occasionally been reported after rubella vaccine. Very rarely neurological symptoms have been reported but a causal relationship has not been established.

11.4.2   Serious reactions following rubella immunisation should be reported to the Committee on Safety of Medicines using the yellow card system.

11.5   Contraindications

(i)   Rubella vaccine should not be given to a woman known to be pregnant, and pregnancy should be avoided for one month after immunisation but see 11.3.2.

(ii)   Immunisation should be postponed if the patient is suffering from a febrile illness until recovery is complete.

(iii)   The vaccine should not be administered to patients receiving high dose corticosteroid (see 3.2.1 iv) or immunosuppressive treatment including general radiation; or to those suffering from malignant conditions of the reticulo-endothelial system such as lymphoma, leukaemia, Hodgkin's disease or where the normal immunological mechanism may be impaired as, for example, in hypogammaglobulinaemia.

(iv)   If it is necessary to administer more than one live virus vaccine at the same time, these may be given simultaneously at different sites unless a combined preparation is used. If not given simultaneously they should be separated by an interval of at least three weeks. A three week interval should be allowed between the administration of rubella vaccine and BCG.

(v)   Rubella vaccine should not be given within three months of an injection of immunoglobulin.

11.5.1   Rubella vaccines contain traces of neomycin and/or polymyxin. Previous anaphylactic reaction to these substances contraindicate rubella immunisation.

11.6   Supplies

Four freeze-dried live vaccines are available, all containing the same strain, Wistar RA 27/3:

Almevax   Evans Medical Tel. 0403 41400
Ervevax   SmithKline Beecham Tel. 0707 325111.
Meruvax   Morson Tel. 0992 467272.
Rubavax   Merieux UK Tel. 0628 785291

11.7   Human normal immunoglobulin (HNIG)

Post-exposure prophylaxis with immunoglobulin does **not** prevent infection in non-immune contacts and is therefore of little value for protection of pregnant women exposed to rubella. It may however reduce the likelihood of clinical symptoms which may possibly reduce the risk to the fetus. It should only be used if termination for confirmed rubella would be unacceptable when it should be given soon after exposure; serological follow-up of recipients is essential.

> Dose: 750mg
> For supplies see 4.10.5.

11.8   Surveillance of CRS and rubella immunisation in pregnancy

11.8.1   Congenital Rubella Syndrome has been included amongst the rare diseases monitored by the British Paediatric Surveillance Unit which sends monthly enquiries to paediatricians.

11.8.2   Any child with congenital rubella defects, or with symptoms suggestive of congenital rubella, or with laboratory evidence of intra-uterine infection without symptoms should also be notified to the National Congenital Rubella Surveillance Scheme:

Ms Pat Tookey
National Congenital Rubella Surveillance Programme
Department of Epidemiology and Biostatistics
Institute of Child Health
30 Guilford Street
London WC1
Tel. 071-242 9789

This Department is also investigating the effects of rubella immunisation in pregnancy. If a woman is given rubella vaccine in pregnancy, or becomes pregnant within one month of immunisation, the Department should be notified as soon as possible. Arrangements will then be made for the appropriate clinical and virological examination of the new-born infant, and for subsequent follow-up.

11.9   Bibliography

Consequences of confirmed maternal rubella at different stages of pregnancy.
Miller E, Cradock-Watson J E, Pollock T M.
Lancet 1982; ii: 781–4.

Rubella vaccination: persistence of antibodies for up to 16 years.
O'Shea S, et al.
BMJ 1982; 285: 253.

Rubella antibody persistence after immunisation.
Chu S Y, Bernier R H, Stewart J A et al.
JAMA 1988; 259: 3133–6.

Rubella vaccination in pregnancy
Tookey P A, Jones G, Miller B H R & Peckham C S
CDR 1991, 1 R 86–88

National Congenital Rubella Surveillance Programme 1.7.71–30.6.84.
Smithells R W, Sheppard S, Holzel H, Dickson A.
BMJ 1985: 291; 40–41.

Rational strategy for rubella vaccination.
Hinman A, Orenstein W, Bart K, Preblud S.
Lancet 1983: i; 39–41.

Some current issues relating to rubella vaccine.
Preblud S.
JAMA 1985; 254 (2): 253–6.

Rubella surveillance to December 1990: A joint report from the PHLS and
National Congenital Rubella Surveillance Programme
Miller E, Waight P A, Verdien J E et al
CDR 1991, I: R 33–37

Congenital rubella in the Asian community in Britain
Miller E, Waight P A, Rousseau S A et al
Br Med J 1990, 301: 1391

Outcome of periconceptional maternal rubella.
Enders G, Nickerl-Packer U, Miller E, Cradock-Watson J E.
Lancet 1988; 11: 1445–6

12   Tuberculosis: BCG immunisation

Please note that this chapter is arranged differently from other chapters in this book. For ease of reference, it is divided into three sections:

 i BCG immunisation policy (paragraphs 12.1 to 12.4).

 ii The tuberculin skin test (paragraphs 12.5 to 12.16).

 iii BCG immunisation technique (paragraphs 12.17 to 12.26).

BCG IMMUNISATION POLICY

12.1   Introduction

12.1.1 Human tuberculosis is caused by infection with *Mycobacterium tuberculosis* or *Mycobacterium bovis* and may affect any part of the body. In the UK, about 75% of new cases involve the respiratory system; non-respiratory forms are more common in immigrant ethnic groups and in those who are immunocompromised. The infection is most commonly acquired by aerosol spread; such transmission is only likely when the index case is sputum smear-positive for the bacillus.

12.1.2 The incidence of tuberculosis in the UK declined tenfold between 1948 and 1987 (see Figure 12.1), although high immigration levels, particularly from the Indian subcontinent (ISC), slowed the decline in the late 1960's. The decline stopped in 1987, since when just over 5,000 new cases have been notified each year. The incidence varies widely between areas, but is generally higher in areas with a high proportion of the population of ISC ethnic origin. Mortality from tuberculosis decreased rapidly after the introduction of effective chemotherapy and in recent years has been about 7%.

Figure 12.1 shows notifications and deaths from tuberculosis from 1940 to 1991.

12.2   Bacillus Calmette-Guerin (BCG) vaccine

12.2.1 BCG vaccine contains a live attenuated strain derived from *Mycobacterium bovis*. It is now available freeze-dried in rubber-capped vials with diluent in a separate ampoule.

12.2.2 The vaccine gives good protection: in British children efficacy in protecting against tuberculosis has been shown to be greater than 70%, protection lasting at least 15 years with little attrition of effectiveness.

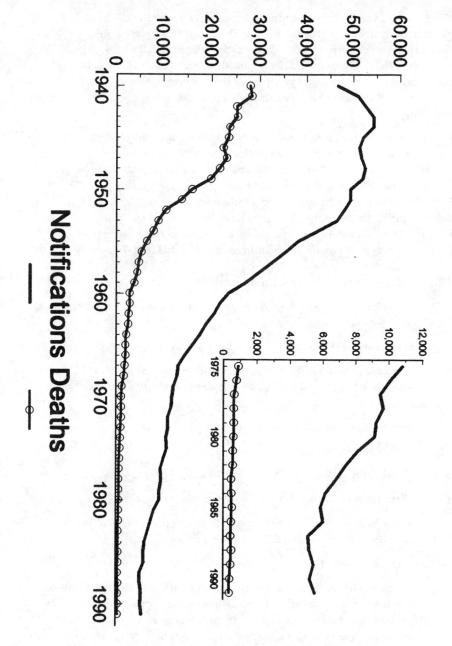

Figure 12.1 Notifications of tuberculosis & deaths (E & W)

12.2.3   BCG vaccine was introduced for general use in the UK in 1953. A national immunisation programme was then started with the aim of immunising all children at age 13 before they left school. By 1958, 35% of children in this age cohort had been immunised and by 1962, 60%. In recent years about 75% of the target group have been immunised each year. A further 5–7% have been already tuberculin positive and therefore exempt from immunisation.

12.2.4   Adverse reactions to BCG vaccine are rare if attention is paid to proper selection of subjects and to the techniques for both tuberculin testing and BCG immunisation. All personnel performing these tests must be properly instructed and observed to be using the correct techniques. The Department of Health has produced a video, for use in teaching sessions, demonstrating the techniques. Copies have been sent to all District Immunisation Coordinators in England, and are also available on free loan (England only) or to buy from the address at the end of this chapter.

12.3   Recommendations for immunisation

12.3.1   The following groups are recommended for immunisation with BCG provided:

a   **successful** BCG immunisation has not previously been carried out, and

b   the tuberculin skin test is negative as defined in paragraphs 12.8.3 and 12.15.2. (Babies up to three months of age may be immunised without prior skin testing.)

c   there are no other contra-indications (see 12.4 below).

12.3.2   Those at **normal risk**:

a   **School children** between the ages of 10 and 13 years.

b   All **students** including those in teacher training colleges.

c   **Newly-born babies, children or adults** where the parents or the individuals themselves request BCG immunisation.

12.3.3   Those at **higher risk**:

a   **Health service staff** who may have contact with infectious patients or their specimens. These comprise doctors, nurses, physiotherapists, radiographers, occupational therapists, technical staff in microbiology and pathology departments including attendants in autopsy rooms, students in all these disciplines, and any others considered to be at high risk. It is particularly important to test and immunise staff working in maternity and paediatric departments.

b **Veterinary and other staff** who handle animal species known to be susceptible to tuberculosis eg simians.

c **Contacts** of cases known to be suffering from active respiratory tuberculosis.

Contacts of a sputum smear positive index case may have a negative tuberculin skin test but be in the early stages of infection because tuberculin sensitivity has not yet developed. Immunisation will do no harm, but if possible should be delayed and the skin test repeated six weeks later. Immunisation is then carried out only if this second test is negative. If the second skin test is positive, the patient has converted and must be referred for consideration of prophylactic chemotherapy. However, it is better to immunise after the first test than not to immunise at all.

Hiv positive contacts of a smear positive case should be referred for consideration of chemoprophylaxis.

Children under five years of age who are contacts of a smear positive case should be given chemoprophylaxis and then immunised with BCG on completion of the course. Newly born babies who are contacts should have prophylactic isoniazid chemotherapy and the tuberculin test repeated after 3-6 months. If positive, chemotherapy is continued; if negative, BCG vaccine is given provided they are no longer in contact with infectious tuberculosis. Newly born contacts of other cases should be immunised immediately.

d **Immigrants from countries with a high prevalence of tuberculosis, their children and infants wherever born**.

New entrants to the UK from countries where tuberculosis is of high prevalence (eg the Indian Subcontinent) must be tuberculin skin tested as part of the initial screening procedure. Those with positive reactions should be referred for investigation and may require chemoprophylaxis. BCG immunisation should be offered immediately to those who are tuberculin negative, and it is recommended their infants born subsequently in this country are immunised within a few days of birth. If this is not done, BCG can conveniently be given at two months of age at the same time as the first dose of the routine childhood vaccines.

e **Those intending to stay in Asia, Africa, Central or South America for more than a month**.

12.3.4   Past successful BCG immunisation will have produced a characteristic colourless, flat, circular scar (usually on the upper arm or lateral aspect of the thigh) which may be supported by a history of immunisation.

Subjects who give a history of previous BCG immunisation should only be reimmunised if there is no characteristic scar **and** they are tuberculin negative.

12.4   Contraindications

12.4.1   BCG vaccine should **NOT** be given to subjects:

a   Receiving corticosteroid or other immunosuppressive treatment including general radiation (see paragraph 3.2 (iii), (iv), (v) on general contraindications to immunisation).

b   Suffering from a malignant condition such as lymphoma, leukaemia, Hodgkin's disease or other tumour of the reticuloendothelial system.

c   In whom the normal immunological mechanism may be impaired, as in hypogammaglobulinaemia.

d   Who are HIV positive (see 3.4 and 12.4.2).

e   Who are pregnant. Although no harmful effects on the fetus have been observed from BCG immunisation during pregnancy, it is wise to avoid immunisation in the early stages and if possible to delay until after delivery.

f   With positive sensitivity tests to tuberculin protein.

g   With pyrexia.

h   With generalised septic skin conditions (but if eczema exists, an immunisation site should be chosen that is free from skin lesions).

12.4.2   BCG should **NOT** be given to symptomatic HIV positive individuals. In areas where the risk of tuberculosis is low, such as the UK, it is recommended that BCG is withheld from all subjects known or suspected to be HIV positive, including infants born to HIV positive mothers.

12.4.3   BCG vaccine may be given concurrently with another live vaccine, but if they are not given at the same time, an interval of at least three weeks should be allowed between such vaccines, whichever is given first. No further immunisation should be given for at least three months in the arm used for BCG immunisation because of the risk of regional lymphadenitis.

12.4.4   When BCG is given to infants, there is no need to delay the primary immunisations, which include polio vaccine, because the latter viruses replicate in the intestine to induce local immunity as well as serum antibodies, and three doses are given.

THE TUBERCULIN SKIN TEST

12.5 Introduction

A tuberculin skin test must be carried out before BCG immunisation. The only exception to this rule is infants up to three months old who may be immunised without a prior test. The test assesses the individuals' sensitivity to tuberculin protein; a positive test implies past infection or past successful immunisation and such people should not be given BCG. Those with strongly positive tests may have active disease and need to be referred to a chest clinic for consideration of further investigation and treatment.

12.6 Tuberculin testing techniques

12.6.1   There are several techniques for tuberculin skin testing. All the common ones have been considered for their reliability, ease of use and safety and only two are recommended for general use: the Mantoux test and the Heaf test. It is strongly recommended that one of these two techniques is used.

12.6.2   Both these tests use Purified Protein Derivative (PPD) which users can obtain from their District Health Authority or Health Board free of charge (see 12.24). The various preparations of PPD are described in 12.7. Care must be taken to ensure that the dilution of PPD used is that specified for the particular technique.

12.6.3   Careful attention must be given to the precautions described for each test to prevent any risk of cross-infection.

12.7 Purified protein derivative

12.7.1   Tuberculin Purified Protein Derivative is a sterile preparation made from the heat-treated products of growth and lysis of the mycobacterium. Several strengths of PPD are available and it is very important that the correct solution is used.

12.7.2   All tuberculin PPD must be stored between 2°C and 8°C (never frozen) and protected from light. Once an ampoule is opened, its contents should be used within one hour and not retained beyond that session. PPD tends to adsorb onto syringe surfaces and should therefore be used within 30 minutes after the syringe is filled. Note that PPD may persist on the surface of any non-disposable syringe and on the endplate and needles of the standard Heaf gun, both of which need careful cleaning subsequently.

Strength units/ml	Dilution of PPD	Units in dose of 0.1 ml	Main use
100,000	–	10,000	Heaf (multiple puncture) test **only**
1,000	1 in 100	100	For special diagnostic purposes **only**
100	1 in 1,000	10	Mantoux test (routine)
10	1 in 10,000	1	Mantoux test (special)

12.8 The Mantoux test

12.8.1 The PPD preparation for routine use in the Mantoux test (dilution 100 units/ml) is supplied in ampoules containing 1.0ml. The contents of an ampoule will therefore be sufficient for five or six texts. For tests in patients in whom tuberculosis is suspected, or who are known to be hypersensitive to tuberculin, a dilution of 10 units/ml should be used. This dilution is not supplied routinely through health authorities and should be ordered direct from Evans Medical or through a retail or wholesale pharmacist.

12.8.2 The Mantoux test is performed using a 1ml syringe and a short bevel 25 gauge (0.5 × 10mm) or 26 gauge (0.45 × 10mm) needle. A separate syringe and needle must be used for each subject to prevent cross-infection.

12.8.3 The test is normally performed on the upper third of the flexor surface of the forearm. The site is cleaned if necessary with spirit and allowed to dry. 0.1ml of tuberculin PPD dilution 100 units/ml is injected **intradermally** so that a bleb (peau d'orange) is produced typically of 7mm diameter. The results should be read 48 to 72 hours later, but a valid reading can usually be obtained up to 96 hours. A positive result consists of transverse induration of at least 5mm diameter following injection of 0.1ml PPD 100 units/ml. 0–4mm induration is negative, 5-14mm is equivalent to a Heaf Grade 2, and 15mm or more, strongly positive (Heaf Grade 3 or 4).

See inside back cover for examples of Heaf test responses

12.9 The multiple puncture test (Heaf test)

12.9.1 This test was conventionally performed with a reusable Heaf multiple puncture apparatus (commonly known as a Heaf gun) which requires disinfection between subjects. Concern that blood borne infections such as hepatitis B and HIV might be transferred via this apparatus should the recommended disinfection procedure not be strictly adhered to, has led to the development of a disposable head apparatus which is now recommended as the preferred method for Heaf testing. It is particularly suitable for the school's BCG programme when multiple tests are performed in one session.

12.9.2   The new apparatus should not be confused with the earlier alternative version of the Heaf gun which had a magnetic head which held a replaceable six point steel-plate. The steel-plate was either discarded or sterilised for re-use. Studies showed a high false negative rate for this technique and the magnetic head itself could become contaminated with body fluids. **Use of this device is not recommended**. Some older Heaf guns had side grips, and these also are not recommended.

12.9.3   Concentrated PPD 100,000 units/ml is used for the Heaf test. This strength is only used for Heaf testing. It is supplied in packs of five ampoules of 1.0ml, each ampoule normally being sufficient for 5-6 tests.

12.10   The standard reusable Heaf gun

12.10.1   The apparatus consists of a needle block of six needles attached to a firing mechanism and handle. The six needles are fired through corresponding holes in the end plate.

12.10.2   Before use the Heaf gun should be checked carefully to ensure that the needles are sharp, clean and not displaced in their retaining plate. It is good practice to replace needles every six months if the gun is in regular use. Periodic servicing of the gun by the manufacturer is also recommended.

12.10.3   The puncture depth of the needles is adjustable and should be set to 2mm for adults and children aged two years or more, and 1mm for children under two years.

12.11   Disinfection of the Heaf gun

12.11.1   The gun must be disinfected before every test and at the end of a testing session and it is essential that the user personally observes this being done. If a sufficient number of spare heads is available, the use of a replacement autoclaved head for each patient is a satisfactory alternative.

12.11.2   The disinfection procedure recommended below is virucidal as long as it is strictly adhered to. It uses highly flammable spirit and proper precautions are needed to prevent fire hazard. The disinfection procedure requires an interval of three minutes or more between consecutive tests with any one instrument. Therefore at least three guns should be available for each team and they should be disinfected and used in rotation. This will sustain a testing rate of 60 subjects an hour with the required interval for disinfection and cooling.

12.11.3   Disinfection is a three stage process:

a   The end of the instrument is immersed in Industrial Methylated Spirit BP to a depth that totally covers the end plate and the needles but does not wet the body of the gun (about 1cm). This should be done in a substantial heavy vessel which will support the gun and ensure immersion at the correct depth for at least two minutes. Industrial methylated spirit is a colourless preparation containing 95% ethyl alcohol adulterated with wood naphtha which will burn readily. Note that this is a volatile liquid that may create a highly flammable vapour. It should not be left in an open vessel near a naked flame. Mineralised methylated spirits (the violet preparation sold retail for general use) and Surgical Spirit BP contain only 90% alcohol and other adulterant substances that may inhibit flammability. They are not satisfactory.

b   The gun is withdrawn from the spirit and held at an angle of 45° to the vertical with the end plate directed upwards. The spirit is set alight by momentary contact with a flame from which the gun is removed on ignition. The spirit is allowed to burn until the flame goes out.

c   Cooling. It is essential to allow adequate time – a minimum of 30 seconds – for the gun to cool, but ensure that the needles do not become contaminated prior to use.

12.12   Maintenance of the Heaf gun

The apparatus requires thorough cleaning after each session. The needles should be scrubbed with a stiff brush using a hot soap or detergent solution and rinsed with distilled water. The needles must be checked to see whether they are becoming blunt or slipping in the retaining plate. Periodic servicing by the manufacturer is recommended.

12.13   The disposable head apparatus

12.13.1   This equipment avoids the need for the disinfection, cleansing and maintenance required for the standard Heaf apparatus. It therefore ensures that no cross infection can occur between subjects and also avoids the possibility of needles becoming blunt and tuberculin building up on needles which are reused.

12.13.2   The disposable heads attach by a magnet to a new simplified handle. Six standard steel needles are retained in a plastic base which is enclosed in an outer plastic case with holes corresponding to the needles. The needles protrude only after actuation and then remain protruding so that it is easy to detect and discard ones which have been fired. The heads are prepacked and sterile.

12.13.3   There are three versions of the disposable head:

i   **White** – this is the standard version for tuberculin testing in adults and children two years and over. The needles protrude 2mm on firing.

ii   **Blue** – for tuberculin testing children under two years. Needles protrude 1mm.

iii   **Red** – this version contains 18 needles for giving BCG by the percutaneous multiple puncture technique and must never be used for Heaf ⸙ testing.

12.14   Performing the Heaf test

12.14.1   The recommended site for testing is on the flexor surface of the left forearm at the junction of the upper third with the lower two thirds, avoiding any eczematous areas. Cleansing the skin is only necessary if it is visibly dirty, in which case spirit should be used but must be allowed to dry completely before the test.

12.14.2   Tuberculin 100,000 units/ml should be withdrawn from the ampoule by needle and syringe and after detaching the needle a small quantity of solution should be dropped directly from the syringe onto the skin at the standard test site. Ensure that there is sufficient tuberculin to disperse over an area of skin just greater than the diameter of the perforated head of the unit. (If using the disposable head apparatus, remember the head is wider than the standard gun). The head of the apparatus should be used to disperse the tuberculin over an area of skin just greater than the area of the head. If using the conventional gun, check that the gun is at the correct setting. The end plate should then be applied firmly and evenly to the area of skin covered by the tuberculin and pressure applied to the handle until the clicking firing mechanism operates. Do not apply further pressure after this, and withdraw the apparatus.

12.14.3   **If using the disposable head apparatus, check that the correct head is being used.** Apply the apparatus firmly and evenly to the tuberculin covered skin and press on the handle until a click occurs, indicating that the needles have been fired. Do not press further after this, but remove the apparatus from the skin, remove the tuberculin head from the handle by holding the outer rim and discard the head into a 'sharps' bin.

12.14.4   Wipe off any excess tuberculin from the skin and observe the presence of **six** puncture marks. If these are not present the test has not been adequately applied. Advise the subject that the arm may be wetted and washed normally but perfumes and other cosmetics should not be applied.

Instructions should be given to the subject to return to have the test read. Ideally this should be at seven days but the test can be read between three and 10 days.

12.15 Interpretation of the Heaf test

12.15.1   The reaction is graded 0–4 according to the degree of induration produced (erythema alone should be ignored). The results should be recorded as a number and not merely as positive or negative.

12.15.2   Grade 0 – no induration at the puncture sites.
Grade 1 – discrete induration at 4 or more needle sites.
Grade 2 -induration around each needle site merging with the next, forming a ring of induration but with a clear centre.
Grade 3 – the centre of the reaction becomes filled with induration to form one uniform circle of induration 5–10mm wide.
Grade 4 – solid induration over 10mm wide. Vesiculation or ulceration may also occur.

12.15.3   Grades 0 and 1 are regarded as negative. Individuals who have not previously received BCG immunisation may be offered immunisation in the absence of contraindications. Those who give a history of previous BCG should only be reimmunised if there is no evidence of a characteristic scar.

12.15.4   Those with a grade 2 reaction (or a Mantoux response of induration of diameter 5–14mm following injection of 0.1ml PPD 100 units/ml) are positive. They are hypersensitive to tuberculin protein and should not be given BCG vaccine. When the immunisation is performed as part of a routine health prevention programme such as the schools programme, no further action is required. In other circumstances (eg immigrants, contacts of tuberculosis etc) subjects with a grade 2 reaction who have not previously had a BCG immunisation should be referred to a chest clinic.

12.15.5   All those who show a strongly positive reaction to tuberculin (grade 3 or 4 or a Mantoux response with induration of at least 15mm diameter following 0.1ml PPD 100 units/ml) should be referred for further investigation and supervision (which may include prophylactic chemotherapy). This includes subjects previously immunised with BCG.

See inside back cover for examples of Heaf test responses.

12.16 Factors affecting the tuberculin test

12.16.1   The reaction to tuberculin protein may be suppressed by the following factors:

a glandular fever;
b viral infections in general, including those of the upper respiratory tract;
c live viral vaccines;
d Hodgkins disease;
e sarcoidosis;
f corticosteroid therapy;
g immunosuppressing diseases, including HIV.

12.16.2 Subjects who have a negative test but who may have had an upper respiratory tract or other viral infection at the time of testing should be retested 2-3 weeks after clinical recovery before being given BCG. Tuberculin testing should not be carried out within three weeks of receiving a live viral vaccine. Immunisation programmes should be arranged so that tuberculin testing is carried out before live viral vaccines are given.

12.16.3 The following factors may also affect the consistency of tuberculin testing or add to its variability:

i tester/reader variation. Even in the best controlled trials there can be a difference of up to 16% between the results of one tester or reader against another. It is essential therefore to minimise these differences by strictly adhering to the techniques described.

ii Skin thickness and reactivity vary in different areas of the body. The tests should therefore always be given at the recommended site.

iii There is some variability in the time at which a test develops its maximum response. For a given test the majority of subjects will be positive at a given time. A few however may have their maximum response just before or after the standard time and their tuberculin reaction could be misinterpreted if read only at the standard time interval.

iv Repeat testing at one site may alter the reactivity either by hypo- or more often hypersensitising the skin. In such instances a changed response at subsequent testing may reflect local changes in sensitivity only.

v Tuberculin adsorption. Tuberculin can adsorb onto materials. Once it has been drawn into a syringe, it should be used within 30 minutes otherwise there may be a deterioration in the tuberculin.

vi Age. There is a tendency for the tuberculin response to diminish with increasing age of the subject.

BCG IMMUNISATION

12.17 Introduction

It is recommended that BCG vaccine be administered intradermally using a separate tuberculin syringe and needle for each subject. **Jet injectors should not be used**. The percutaneous route (using a modified Heaf gun) is an acceptable alternative to the intradermal method for neonates, infants and very young children **only**. **It is not recommended for older children, teenagers and adults**. 18–20 needles are required and BCG vaccine prepared specifically for percutaneous use (see paragraph 22.3 below).

12.18 Preparation of the vaccine

12.18.1   Freeze-dried vaccine is supplied to NHS users without charge by Health Authorities/Health Boards who order it from the appropriate government Health Department (see 12.24 below).

12.18.2   The freeze-dried vaccine should be protected from light, stored between 2° and 8°C and never frozen. It has a shelf life of 12-18 months and should not be used after the expiry date stated on the label.

12.18.3   The multidose vial of vaccine should be diluted as instructed on the package insert using aseptic precautions, a syringe and suitable large needle. Do not shake it to mix. The needle may be left in situ for subsequent withdrawal of vaccine. Once made up the vaccine should be used within two hours. Any unused reconstituted vaccine should be discarded at the end of the session.

12.18.4   For tuberculosis contacts on isoniazid prophylactic therapy, isoniazid-resistant BCG vaccine is available and should be ordered by the user direct from the manufacturer, Evans Medical Ltd, or through a pharmaceutical wholesaler.

12.19 Immunisation Technique

12.19.1   The recommended site for giving the vaccine is at the insertion of the deltoid muscle near the middle of the left upper arm. Sites higher on the arm are more likely to lead to keloid formation, the tip of the shoulder particularly. In girls, for cosmetic reasons, the upper and lateral surface of the thigh may be preferred.

Figure 12.2 shows the recommended site for BCG immunisation.

12.19.2   The vaccine must be given strictly intradermally with a fresh needle

Figure 12.2   The site and technique for BCG immunisation

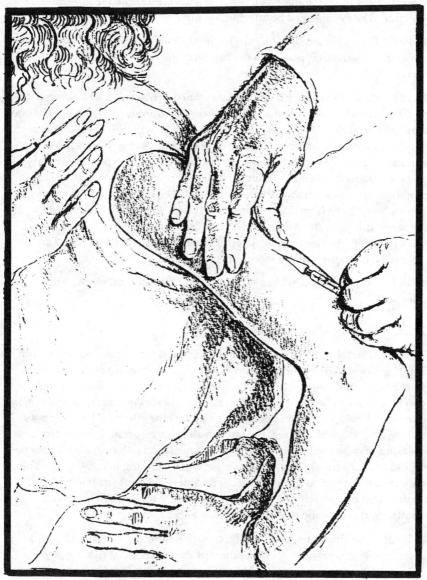

Margaret Maskew

Tuberculosis

and syringe for each subject. The dose is 0.1ml (0.05ml for infants under three months). This should be drawn into a tuberculin syringe and a ⅜" 25g (0.5 × 10mm) or 26g (0.45 × 10mm) short bevelled needle attached to give the injection. The needle must be attached firmly with the bevel uppermost.

12.19.3   The upper arm must be approximately 45° to the body. This can be achieved if the hand is placed on the hip with the arm abducted from the body.

12.19.4   If the skin is dirty it should be swabbed with spirit and allowed to dry. The operator stretches the skin between the thumb and forefinger of one hand and with the other slowly inserts the needle, with the bevel upwards, for about 2mm into the superficial layers of the dermis almost parallel with the surface. The needle can usually be seen through the epidermis. A correctly given intradermal injection results in a tense blanched raised bleb (peau d'orange) and considerable resistance is felt when the fluid is being injected. A bleb typically of 7mm diameter follows 0.1ml injection. If little resistance is felt when injecting and a diffuse swelling occurs as opposed to a tense blanched bleb, the needle is too deep. The needle should be removed and reinserted elsewhere before more vaccine is given.

12.19.5   The subject must always be advised of the normal reaction to the injection.

12.20   Immunisation reaction

12.20.1   Normally a local reaction develops at the immunisation site within two to six weeks, beginning as a small papule which increases in size for a few weeks widening into a circular area up to 7mm in diameter with scaling, crusting and occasional bruising. Occasionally a shallow ulcer up to 10mm in diameter develops. It is not necessary to protect the site from becoming wet during washing and bathing, but should any oozing occur, a temporary dry dressing may be used until a scab forms. It is essential that air should not be excluded. If absolutely essential an impervious dressing may be applied but only for a short period (for example, to permit swimming) as it may delay healing and cause a larger scar. The lesion slowly subsides over several months and eventually heals leaving only a small scar.

12.20.2   After immunisation with BCG vaccine there is a high tuberculin conversion rate and further observation of those at normal risk is not necessary, nor is further tuberculin testing recommended. However, in large immunisation programmes, some check should be made for adverse reactions six weeks or so later, possibly on a sample basis.

12.20.3   After immunisation of those at **higher risk**, subsequent inspection of the site is a matter for clinical discretion except for **health-care staff judged to be at high risk,** in whom the site of immunisation should be inspected six weeks later to confirm that a satisfactory reaction has occurred. Reactions should be recorded by measuring the transverse diameter in mm. A scar of 4mm or more is satisfactory. Only those who show no reaction to BCG require a post-BCG tuberculin test, after which anyone who is still tuberculin negative should be reimmunised. If after reimmunisation there is still no evidence of a satisfactory reaction or of conversion to a positive tuberculin test, consideration should be given to moving the subject to work not involving exposure to patients with TB or with tuberculous material.

12.21   Adverse reactions to BCG

12.21.1   Severe injection site reactions, large ulcers and abscesses are most commonly caused by faulty injection technique where part or all of the dose is administered too deeply (subcutaneously instead of intradermally). The immunisation of individuals who are tuberculin positive may also give rise to such reactions. To avoid these, doctors and nurses who carry out tuberculin skin tests and administer BCG vaccine **must** be trained in the interpretation of the results of tuberculin tests as well as in the technique of intradermal injection with syringe and needle.

12.21.2   Keloid formation at the injection site is a not uncommon, but largely avoidable, complication of BCG immunisation. Some sites are more prone to keloid formation than others and those immunising should adhere to the two sites recommended in this chapter (the mid-upper arm or the thigh). Most experience has been gained in the use of the upper arm and it is known that the risk of keloid formation is increased manyfold when the injection is given at a site higher than the **insertion of the deltoid muscle near the middle of the upper arm (see 19.4 and figure).**

12.21.3   Apart from these injection site reactions, other complications following BCG immunisation are rare and mostly consist of adenitis with or without suppuration and discharge. A minor degree of adenitis may occur in the weeks following immunisation and should not be regarded as a complication. Very rarely a lupoid type of local lesion has been reported. A few cases of widespread dissemination of the injected organisms have been reported and anaphylactic reactions can occur.

12.21.4   It is important that all complications should be recorded and reported to a chest physician. Serious or unusual complications (including abscess and keloid scarring) should be reported to the Committee on Safety of Medicines using the yellow card system, and techniques reviewed. Every effort should be made to recover and identify the causative organism from any lesion constituting a serious complication.

12.22 Percutaneous BCG Immunisation by the Multiple Puncture Technique

12.22.1   BCG immunisation by intradermal injection, using a separate needle and syringe for every subject, is the only recommended method for older children, teenagers and adults. However, this technique can be difficult in infants and very young children. In these latter groups **only**, percutaneous BCG immunisation by multiple-puncture technique is an acceptable alternative.

12.22.2   The site of injection is over the insertion of the deltoid muscle as previously described. 18–20 needle punctures, with 2mm skin penetration at a pressure of 5–9lb, are required (see 12.24 below for suppliers).

12.22.3   Only percutaneous BCG vaccine, which has 50–250 colony forming units/vial, should be used. Users can obtain this from their Health Authority/ Health Board free of charge.

12.23 Record keeping and surveillance

12.23.1   It is important that records be maintained to show the result of tuberculin skin testing, whether the subject had previously received BCG, and whether or not BCG was subsequently given. These records should show who administered the skin test or vaccine, the batch number of the vaccine, and who recorded the result or lesion. Particular attention should be paid to unusual or severe reactions. Such records should be kept for at least 10 years.

12.23.2   The results of tuberculin skin tests and of BCG immunisation of hospital staff (including students) should be recorded on appropriate records. If staff or students move to another hospital or to another training school, the record cards should be transferred to the occupational health unit.

12.24 Supplies of BCG vaccine and PPD

12.24.1   In England, supplies of freeze-dried BCG vaccine (intradermal and percutaneous) and Tuberculin PPD are distributed to District Health Authorities once a month. DHAs should make the products available to users without charge. Orders for at least one month's requirement should be submitted on the DHAs own order form to reach the Department of Health by the first day of the month preceding the month when the materials are required, eg materials for use in August should be ordered by 1st July. The order should be sent to:

NHS Supplies Authority
Room 222
14 Russell Square
London WC1B 5EP
071-636 6811

12.24.2   In Scotland, the Health Boards order BCG vaccine direct from Vestric as and when required but Tuberculin PPD is distributed to users direct every month and should be ordered from:

The Central Infusion Laboratory
Knightswood Hospital
Glasgow G13 2XG
041-954 8183

12.24.3   In Wales, orders for both BCG vaccine and PPD should be sent monthly by health authorities (as for England) to:

Welsh Health Common Services Authority
Heron House
35–43 Newport Road
Cardiff CF2 1SB
0222-471234 extension 2068

12.24.4   In Northern Ireland, Health and Social Services Boards order both BCG vaccine and PPD from:

Central Services Agency
27 Adelaide Street
Belfast BT2 8FH
0232-324431

12.24.5   Those who require isoniazid-resistant BCG vaccine or non-routine strengths of PPD should order direct from:

Evans Medical Ltd
Distribution Centre
Foster Avenue
Woodside Park Estate
DUNSTABLE Bedfordshire LU5 5TA
0528-476611
Telefax 0582-600421

12.25   A suitable 20 needle modified Heaf gun for percutaneous BCG immunisation is available from Evans Medical, Oxford. The same precautions are required to prevent cross-infection as for Heaf testing. An 18 needle fixed head gun and an 18 needle disposable head for use with the new Bignell 2000 multiple puncture apparatus, are available from Bignell Surgical Instruments, Littlehampton.

12.26   The Department of Health Video

The Department of Health's video 'Heaf Testing and BCG Vaccination: A Practical Guide' (UK 6257) is available to Nursing and Medical Professionals on free loan for five days (in England only) and to purchase for £12.50 inc VAT from CFL Vision, PO Box 35, Wetherby, Yorkshire LS23 7EX, Telephone number 0937 541010 (cheques payable to CFL Vision).

12.27   Bibliography

Tuberculosis and human immunodeficiency virus infection.
Chaisson R E and Slutkin G.
J Infect Dis 1989; 159; 96–100.

National survey of notifications of tuberculosis in England and Wales in 1983.
Tuberculosis and Chest Diseases Unit. Medical Research Council.
BMJ 1985; 291; 658-61.

Tuberculosis among immigrants to England and Wales: a national survey in 1965.
British Tuberculosis Association.
Tubercle 1966; 47; 145–56.

Effectiveness of BCG vaccination in England and Wales in 1983.
Sutherland I and Springett V H.
Tubercle 1987; 68; 81–92.

The prevalence of keloid formation in BCG scars.
Lunn J A and Robson D C.
Personal communication.

The Heaf test: a comparison of two types of Heaf gun.
MacHale E M and O'Shea M E B.
Irish Medical Journal 1987; 80; 400–401.

The tuberculin test in clinical practice: an illustrated guide.
Caplin Maxwell.
Bailliere Tindall, London (1980).

Control and prevention of tuberculosis: an updated Code of Practice. Joint Tuberculosis Committee of the British Thoracic Society. Brit Med J 1990 **300** 995–98.

HIV and routine childhood immunisation
WHO Wkly Epidem Rec 1987 **62** 297–9.

13   Influenza

13.1   Introduction

13.1.1   Influenza is an acute viral disease of the respiratory tract affecting all age groups and characterised by the abrupt onset of fever, chills, headache, myalgia and sometimes prostration. A dry cough is almost invariable and there may be a sore throat. It is usually a self-limiting disease with recovery in two to seven days, but it can be a serious illness. In those with chronic underlying disease, especially if elderly, complications are common and hospitalisation rates high. Mortality is increased, mainly from secondary bacterial pneumonia, but also from the underlying disease. Primary influenzal pneumonia is a rare complication with a high case fatality rate. 3,000–4,000 deaths are attributed to "influenza" even in winters when the incidence is low.

13.1.2   Influenza is highly infectious, spreading rapidly especially in institutions. Epidemics are unpredictable, can evolve rapidly, and are generally associated with a large number of excess deaths mainly among the elderly.

13.1.3   Serological studies show that asymptomatic infection also occurs.

13.1.4   Two types of influenza virus are responsible for most clinical illness, influenza A and influenza B. Outbreaks of infection with influenza A occur most years and these are also the usual cause of epidemics. Influenza B infection tends to occur at intervals of several years.

13.1.5   Influenza A viruses are antigenically labile due to changes in the principal surface antigens, haemagglutinin (H) and neuraminidase (N). Minor changes ("antigenic drift") are seen progressively from season to season. Major changes ("antigenic shift") due to acquisition of a 'new' haemagglutinin occur periodically and are responsible for the emergence of new sub-types to which populations may have little immunity. They can therefore cause epidemics or pandemics.

13.2   Influenza vaccine

13.2.1   Influenza vaccine is prepared each year using virus strains similar to those considered most likely to be circulating in the forthcoming season. Current vaccines are trivalent containing two type A and one type B virus strains, but monovalent vaccines containing the antigens of only one strain of virus may sometimes be produced.

13.2.2   The viruses are highly purified, grown in embryonated hen's eggs and inactivated. Two types are available: "disrupted virus" vaccine contains virus components prepared by treating whole viruses with organic solvents or detergents and then centrifuging. "Surface antigen" vaccine contains highly purified haemagglutinin and neuraminidase antigens prepared from disrupted virus particles. The antigens may be adsorbed onto aluminium hydroxide.

13.2.3   Currently available influenza vaccines give about 70% protection against infection to influenza virus strains related to those in the vaccine. In the elderly, protection against infection may be less, but immunisation of elderly people – especially if they are in residential homes – has been shown to reduce the incidence of bronchopneumonia, hospital admissions and mortality. Protection lasts for about one year and to provide continuing protection, annual immunisation is necessary with vaccine containing the most recent strains.

13.2.4   The vaccines should be stored at 2–8°C and protected from light.

13.3   Recommendations

13.3.1   The aim of influenza immunisation is to protect those who are at increased risk of complications should they develop influenza. Immunisation is therefore strongly recommended for adults and children with any of the following:

a   chronic respiratory disease, including asthma
b   chronic heart disease
c   chronic renal failure .
d   diabetes mellitus and other endocrine disorders
e   immunosuppression due to disease or treatment

13.3.2   Immunisation is also recommended for residents of nursing homes, old peoples' homes and other long stay facilities where rapid spread is likely to follow introduction of infection.

13.3.3   Immunisation of fit children and adults, including health care and other key workers, is not recommended as a routine.

13.3.4   The final decision as to who should be offered immunisation is a matter for the patient's medical practitioner.

13.3.5   Any changes to these recommendations, and details of the composition and doses of each year's vaccines, are issued by the Departments of Health in annual letters from the Chief Medical Officers.

13.3.6   Influenza vaccine may be given at the same time as pneumococcal vaccine, at a different site, **but note that pneumococcal vaccine is given once only**.

13.4   Dosage and Method of Administration

13.4.1   Adults – a single injection of 0.5ml im or sc.
Children aged 4–12 – 0.5ml im, repeated 4–6 weeks later if receiving influenza vaccine for the first time
Children aged 6 months-3 years – 0.25ml im repeated 4–6 weeks later if receiving influenza vaccine for the first time.

13.4.2   All available vaccines are suitable for children aged 4 years and over. The Servier and Merieux products are licensed for use in children from 6 months of age.

13.4.3   The deltoid muscle is the recommended site for adults and older children. For infants and young children the preferred site is the anterolateral aspect of the thigh.

13.4.4   The vaccine should be allowed to reach room temperature before being given.

13.4.5   Antibody levels may take up to 10–14 days to rise. Influenza activity is rarely significant before the end of November, and therefore the ideal time for immunisation is late October/early November.

13.5   Adverse reactions

13.5.1   Influenza vaccine is usually well tolerated apart from occasional soreness at the immunisation site. In rare instances it can, however, cause:

a   Fever, malaise and myalgia beginning 6 to 12 hours after immunisation and lasting up to 48 hours.
b   Immediate reactions such as urticaria, angio-oedema, bronchospasm and anaphylaxis, most likely due to hypersensitivity to residual egg protein.

13.5.2   No association has been found between current vaccine strains and the Guillain-Barré syndrome.

13.5.3   Influenza vaccine contains inactivated virus and cannot cause influenza. Patients should be warned that many other organisms cause respiratory infections during the influenza season and influenza vaccine will not prevent these, otherwise patients may become disillusioned with the vaccine especially in a non epidemic year.

Influenza

13.6   Contraindications

13.6.1   The vaccines are prepared in hens' eggs and should not be given where there is known anaphylactic hypersensitivity to egg products.

13.6.2   The significance of influenza during pregnancy is uncertain. Some evidence from past pandemics suggested that influenza in pregnancy might be associated with increased risk of maternal mortality and congenital malformations and leukaemia in the children; other studies have not supported this. There is no evidence that influenza vaccine prepared from inactivated virus causes damage to the fetus. However, it should not be given during pregnancy unless there is a specific indication.

13.7   Amantadine in the prevention of influenza

13.7.1   Amantadine hydrochloride is an effective antiviral agent against influenza A and may be used prophylactically to control an outbreak proven to be due to, or occurring during an epidemic of, influenza A in the following circumstances:

a   For unimmunised patients in the 'at risk' groups for two weeks while the vaccine takes effect.

b   For patients in the 'at risk' groups in whom immunisation is contraindicated, for the duration of the outbreak.

c   For health care workers and other key personnel to prevent disruption of services during an epidemic.

13.7.2   The recommended dose is 100mg daily. Higher doses are associated with more adverse reactions.

13.7.3   Adverse reactions include insomnia, restlessness and anxiety, nausea and anorexia. Epileptic fits have occasionally occurred, mainly in the elderly taking doses higher than 100 mg/day.

13.7.4   Amantadine should not be used indiscriminantly as there is evidence that drug resistant virus may emerge.

13.8   Supplies

Information on current vaccines is given in the latest CMO letter from the Department of Health. Vaccines are available from:

Duphar Tel. 0703 472281
Evans Medical Ltd Tel. 0582 476611
Servier Tel. 0753 662744
Merieux UK Tel. 0628 785291

13.9   Bibliography

Efficacy of Influenza Vaccine in Nursing Homes
Reduction in Illness and Complications during an Influenza A (H_3N_2)
Epidemic
Patriarca P A, Weber J A, Parker R A et al
JAMA, 1985, **253**, 1136–1139.

Influenza Vaccination of Elderly Persons
Reduction in Pneumonia, Influenza Hospitalisations and Deaths
Barker W H and Mullooly J P
JAMA, 1980, **244**, 2547–2549.

Hidden Influenza Deaths
Curwen M, Dunnell K, Ashley J
BMJ, 1990, **300**, 896,

Simultaneous Administration of Influenza and Pneumococcal Vaccines
De Stefano F, Goodman R A, Noble G R et al
JAMA, 1982, **F247**, 2551–2554

Association of Influenza Immunisation with Reduction in Mortality in an
Elderly Population. A Prospective Study
Gross P A, Quinnan G V, Rodstein M et al
Arch Int Med, 1988, **148**, 562–565.

Current Status of amantadine and rimantadine as anti-influenza A agents.
World Health Organisation Memorandum. Bull WHO 1985 **63** 51–6.

Influenza

14 Pneumococcal Infection

14.1 Introduction

14.1.1   Invasive pneumococcal disease (pneumonia, bacteraemia and meningitis) is a major cause of morbidity and mortality, especially among the very young, the elderly, those with an absent or non-functioning spleen and those with impaired immunity. Pneumococcal pneumonia is estimated to affect 1/1000 adults each year and has a mortality of 10–20%. The pneumococcus is the commonest pathogen in pneumonias acquired in the community. Between 1975 and 1980 the pneumococcus was also responsible for 9% of bacteraemias reported to CDSC, and the proportion has been rising since. Between 1980 and 1984 one fifth of 7,605 cases of bacterial meningitis reported to CDSC were pneumococcal in origin, although a proportion would have been recurrent infections associated with abnormalities such as fractures of the skull.

14.1.2   *Streptococcus pneumoniae* (the pneumococcus) is an encapsulated Gram positive coccus. 84 capsular types have been characterised, of which 8–10 cause two thirds of the serious infections in adults and about 85% of infections in children. Immunity to infection is complicated, but depends greatly on type specific anti-capsular antibodies. However there is no absolute antibody level which might be called protective.

14.2 Pneumococcal Vaccine

14.2.1   Pneumococcal vaccine is a polyvalent vaccine containing 25 microgrammes of purified capsular polysaccharide from each of 23 capsular types of pneumococcus which together account for 90% of the pneumococcal isolates causing serious infection in Britain. It is supplied in a single dose vial.

14.2.2   Most healthy adults develop a good antibody response to a single dose of the vaccine. Antibody response is not so reliable in young children, those with immunological impairment and those being treated with immunosuppressive therapy.

14.2.3   Many studies of efficacy have found it difficult to reach firm conclusions, but overall efficacy in preventing pneumococcal pneumonia is probably 60–70%. Efficacy is less in young children and in those with immunosuppression. Vaccine is not effective in children under two years of age. It does not prevent otitis media or exacerbations of chronic bronchitis, and since so much pneumococcal meningitis is in young children and those with skull defects, its scope for preventing this disease is limited. The vaccine has been relatively ineffective in patients with multiple myeloma, Hodgkins and non-Hodgkins lymphoma, especially during treatment, and chronic alcoholism.

14.2.4   Antibody levels usually begin to wane after about five years, but may decline more rapidly in asplenic patients and children with nephrotic syndrome.

14.3   Recommendations

14.3.1   Pneumococcal vaccine should be considered for all those aged over two years in whom pneumococcal infection is likely to be more common and/or dangerous, ie those with:

i   Homozygous sickle cell disease.

ii   Asplenia or severe dysfunction of the spleen.

iii   Chronic renal disease or nephrotic syndrome.

iv   Immunodeficiency or immunosuppression due to disease or treatment, including HIV infection at all stages.

v   Chronic heart disease.

vi   Chronic lung disease.

vii   Chronic liver disease including cirrhosis.

viii   Diabetes mellitus.

14.3.2   Where possible, the vaccine should be given two weeks before splenectomy, together with advice about the increased risk of pneumococcal infection, and before courses of chemotherapy. Additional penicillin prophylaxis is advisable for children with sickle cell disease or other splenic dysfunction.

14.3.3   It is recommended that opportunities are taken to immunise 'at risk' patients who have not previously been immunised:

i   at routine GP or hospital consultations;

ii   on discharge after hospital admission;

iii   when immunising against influenza.

14.3.4   Pneumococcal vaccine may be given at the same time as influenza vaccine, at a different site, but note that whereas influenza vaccine must be given annually, pneumococcal vaccine is given once only.

Pneumococcal Infection

14.4 Dose and Administration

A single dose of 0.5ml is given subcutaneously or intramuscularly into the deltoid muscle or lateral aspect of the mid thigh. Intradermal injection may cause severe local reaction. The vaccine must not be given intravenously.

14.5 Reimmunisation

Reimmunisation is not normally advised (see 14.6.2) except, after 5–10 years, in individuals in whom antibody levels are likely to have declined more rapidly such as those with no spleen, with splenic dysfunction or with nephrotic syndrome.

14.6 Adverse Reactions

14.6.1   Mild soreness and induration at the site of injection and, less commonly, a low grade fever may occur.

14.6.2   Reimmunisation with the earlier 12 and 14-valent vaccines produced more severe reactions in some recipients, especially if less than five years had elapsed since the first injection. Reactions correlated with high levels of circulating antibodies. Caution is therefore advised when considering reimmunisation with the 23-valent vaccine.

14.7 Contra-indications

14.7.1   Pneumococcal vaccine should not be given during an acute infection. The vaccine has not been evaluated, and should therefore not be given in pregnancy.

14.7.2   Reimmunisation within three years of a previous dose of pneumococcal vaccine is contra-indicated.

14.8 Storage

Vaccine should be stored unopened at 2–8°C and discarded after the expiry date.

14.9 Supplies

Pneumococcal vaccine is supplied by Merck, Sharpe and Dohme Ltd, Hertford Road, Hoddesdon, Herts EN11 9BU, Tel: 0992 467272.

14.10 Bibliography

Community-acquired Pneumonia in Adults in British Hospitals in 1982-83: A survey of Aetiology, Mortality, Prognostic Factors and Outcome.
Br Thoracic Society Research Committee,
Q J Med 1987 **62** 195–220.

Hospital Study of Adult Community-acquired Pneumonia.
MacFarlane J T, Ward M J, Finch R D, Macrae A D,
Lancet 1982, **ii**, 255–8.

Pneumococcal Infections.
Mufson M A,
JAMA 1981 **246** 1942–8.

Resolving the Pneumococcal Vaccine Controversy: Are there Alternatives to Randomised Clinical Trials.
Clemens J D, Shapiro E D,
Rev Inf Dis 1984, **6** 589–600.

Pneumococcal Infection

15 Hepatitis A

15.1 Introduction

15.1.1 Hepatitis A is transmitted by the faecal-oral route. Person-to person spread is the most common method of transmission although contaminated food or drink may sometimes be involved. The incubation period is about 15–40 days and the disease is generally mild or sub-clinical. Asymptomatic disease is common in children and severity tends to increase with age. Occasional cases of fulminating hepatitis may occur but there is no chronic carrier state and little likelihood of chronic liver damage.

15.1.2 Over 80% of cases are contracted in the UK and, whilst the majority of these are sporadic, outbreaks do occur. Laboratory reports of hepatitis A to the Public Health Laboratory Service fell from a peak of just over 4000 reports from England in 1982 to just over 2000 reports per year between 1983 and 1986. Since 1986 the number of reports increased each year to 1990 when over 7500 cases were reported. Whilst there was a small decrease in 1991 the number of reports received was still in excess of 7000 and reports have increased again in the first few months of 1992.

15.1.3 The prevalence of hepatitis A in countries outside Northern and Western Europe, North America, Australia and New Zealand is higher than in the UK and travellers to these countries may be at increased risk of contracting hepatitis A.

15.2 Vaccine

15.2.1 Hepatitis A vaccine has recently been licensed for use in the United Kingdom. It is a formaldehyde-inactivated vaccine prepared from the HM 175 strain of hepatitis A virus (HAV) grown in human diploid cells and supplied as a suspension in pre-filled syringes.

15.2.2 The vaccine should be stored at 2–8°C but not frozen. The shelf-life is two years and it should be protected from light. It should not be diluted or mixed with other vaccines in the same syringe.

15.2.3 Immunogenicity studies show that levels of neutralising antibody produced after a primary course of two doses of vaccine administered intramuscularly two weeks to one month apart are well in excess of those found after administration of HNIG. The primary course produces anti-HAV antibodies which persist for at least one year and antibody persistence can be prolonged by administration of a booster dose of vaccine 6 to 12 months after the initial course.

Hepatitis A

15.2.4   Human normal immunoglobulin may be administered at the same time as vaccine if immediate protection is required. Studies suggest that this results in lower titres of antibody and this may affect the duration of protection.

15.3   Recommendations

15.3.1   Travellers

The vaccine is an alternative to human normal immunoglobulin (see 15.9.c) for frequent adult travellers to areas of high or moderate HAV endemicity or those staying for more than three months in such areas. Immunisation is **not** considered necessary for those travelling to Northern or Western Europe (including Spain, Portugal and Italy), to North America, Australia or New Zealand.

Where practicable, testing for antibodies to hepatitis A virus prior to immunisation may be worthwhile in those aged fifty years or over, those born in areas of high or moderate HAV endemicity and those who have a history of jaundice.

Similar considerations will apply to military personnel being posted or likely to be posted abroad.

15.3.2   Occupational exposure

There is little UK data on the risk of hepatitis A in relation to occupation. Epidemiological studies may help to clarify risk groups.

There is no evidence that health care workers as a group are at increased risk of hepatitis A. Outbreaks of hepatitis A have been associated with residential institutions for the mentally handicapped. Transmission may occur more readily in such institutions and immunisation of staff and inmates should be considered in the light of local circumstances. Similar considerations may apply in other institutions where standards of personal hygiene are poor.

Infection in young children is likely to be clinically silent and those working in day care centres and other settings with children who are not yet toilet-trained may be at increased risk of infection. The risk of transmission to staff can be minimised by careful attention to personal hygiene but local circumstances, eg local community outbreaks, may prompt consideration of immunisation of members of staff.

National surveillance data indicates an occupational risk of infection for sewage workers and immunisation should be considered in this group.

Military and diplomatic personnel should be considered at increased risk of infection inasmuch as their employment involves residence in areas of moderate and high HAV endemicity.

There is no evidence to suggest that food packagers or food handlers in the United Kingdom have been associated with HAV transmission sufficiently often to justify their immunisation as a routine measure.

15.3.3   Outbreaks of hepatitis A in homosexual males have been reported in the United Kingdom but there is currently no data to support routine immunisation in this group nor in drug abusers.

15.3.4   Recommendations on the use of hepatitis A vaccine in outbreaks or in contacts of cases cannot yet be made as data are not yet available on its effectiveness, alone or in combination with human normal immunoglobulin, in post-exposure prophylaxis (see 15.9). Further guidance on the management of outbreaks should be sought from the Consultant in Communicable Disease Control or from the PHLS Communicable Disease Surveillance Centre.

15.4   Route of administration and dosage

15.4.1   The immunisation regimen consists of two doses of vaccine spaced two weeks to one month apart. Antibodies produced in response to this primary course persist for at least one year. A booster dose at 6–12 months after the primary course results in more persistent antibodies.

The vaccine should be given intramuscularly in the deltoid region. It should not be given in the gluteal region because vaccine efficacy may be reduced nor should it be administered intravenously, intradermally or subcutaneously.

15.4.2   Dosage

The adult dose is 720 ELISA units (1 ml).

No paediatric dose has yet been established and vaccine is not yet licensed for use in children and adolescents less than 16 years of age.

15.5   Adverse reactions

In clinical trials adverse reactions were usually mild and confined to the first few days after immunisation. The most common reactions were mild transient soreness, erythema and induration at the injection site. General symptoms such as fever, malaise, fatigue, headache, nausea and loss of appetite were also reported less frequently.

It is important that adverse reactions should be reported to the Committee on Safety of Medicines by the yellow card system.

15.6 Contraindications

Immunisation should be postponed in individuals suffering from severe febrile infections.

The effect of HAV vaccine on fetal development has not been assessed. Since it is an inactivated vaccine, the risks to the fetus are likely to be negligible but, as with other vaccines in pregnancy, it should not be given unless there is a definite risk of infection.

15.7 Supplies of Hepatitis A Vaccine

Havrix   SmithKline Beecham. Tel. 0707 325111.

15.8 Immunoglobulin

15.8.1   Human normal immunoglobulin (HNIG) offers short-term protection against infection with hepatitis A to those in close contact with cases and to those travelling to areas where infection is more prevalent, particularly if sanitation and food hygiene are likely to be poor.

15.8.2   Although infection is commonly subclinical in young children and severe infection uncommon, the decision to use HNIG may be influenced by the wish to protect parents and other adult contacts. Evidence suggests that, even if HNIG modifies disease rather than preventing infection, it is effective in preventing secondary cases.

15.8.3   There is no evidence associating the administration of intramuscular immunoglobulin with transmission of HIV. Not only does the processing of the plasma from which it is prepared render it safe, but the plasma is derived from screened blood donations.

15.9 Recommendations

Use of HNIG should be considered in the following circumstances:

a   **Contacts of cases of hepatitis A infection.**

Prophylaxis restricted to household and close social contacts may be relatively ineffective in controlling further spread. If given to a wider social group of recent household visitors (kissing contacts and those who have eaten food prepared by the index case) spread may be more effectively prevented.

b   **Outbreaks**

The appropriate approach to prophylaxis should be discussed with the Consultant in Communicable Disease Control.

In schools, consideration should be given to protecting teachers, adult helpers and the children and parents of children in the affected classes.

In closed communities where personal hygiene may be poor, widespread use of HNIG should be considered.

c **Travellers**

Administration of HNIG should be considered in those travelling occasionally and for short periods to countries outside Northern and Western Europe, North America, Australia and New Zealand. Hepatitis A vaccine is likely to be preferable for those aged 16 or over visiting such countries frequently or staying for longer than three months (see 15.3.1).

Where practicable, testing for antibodies to hepatitis A virus prior to immunisation may be worthwhile in those aged fifty years or over, those born in areas of high or moderate HAV endemicity and those who have a history of jaundice.

Human normal immunoglobulin may interfere with the development of active immunity from live virus vaccines. It is therefore wise to administer live virus vaccines at least three weeks before the administration of immunoglobulin. If immunoglobulin has been administered first, then an interval of three months should be observed before administering a live virus vaccine. This does not apply to yellow fever vaccine since HNIG does not contain antibody to this virus. For travellers, if there is insufficient time, the recommended intervals may have to be ignored, especially where oral polio vaccine is concerned. Alternatively, hepatitis A vaccine may be used in these circumstances.

15.10 Dosage

At present, the dosage of HNIG is expressed either by weight (mg) or by volume (ml). 1 ml of a 16% solution contains 160 mg.

Age	Low dose For travel lasting 2 months or less	High dose For travel lasting 3–5 months and for contacts
Under 10y	125 mg	250 mg
10y and over	250 mg	500 mg
or		
All ages	0.02–0.04 ml/kg	0.06–0.12 ml/kg

There are two dosage levels. The higher dose is recommended for those at greater risk (ie contacts) and for extended protection (ie those travelling abroad for 3–5 months).

15.11 Supplies

Bio-Products Laboratory Tel. 081-953 6191
Scottish National Blood Transfusion Service
The Laboratories,Belfast City Hospital Tel. 0232 329241

Immuno (Gammabulin), Tel. 0732 458101
Kabi Pharmacia (Kabiglobulin), Tel. 0908 661101

For contacts and the control of outbreaks only:

PHLS Communicable Diseases Surveillance Centre, Tel. 081-200 6868
Public Health Laboratories, England and Wales

Hepatitis A

16   Hepatitis B

16.1   Introduction

16.1.1   Hepatitis B is transmitted parenterally. Transmission most commonly occurs as a result of blood to blood contact, including injury with contaminated sharp instruments and sharing of needles by intravenous drug abusers, following vaginal or anal intercourse or by perinatal transmission from mother to child. Transmission has also rarely followed bites from infected persons. Transfusion-associated infection is now rare and treatment of blood products has eliminated these as sources of infection.

16.1.2   The illness usually has an insidious onset with anorexia, vague abdominal discomfort, nausea and vomiting, sometimes arthralgia and rash, which often progresses to jaundice. Fever may be absent or mild. The severity of the disease ranges from inapparent infections, which can only be detected by liver function tests and/or the presence of serological markers of acute HBV infection (eg HBsAg, antiHBc IgM), to fulminating fatal cases of acute hepatic necrosis. Among cases admitted to hospital the fatality rate is about 1%. The average incubation period is 40–160 days but occasionally can be as long as nine months.

16.1.3   About 2–10% of those infected as adults become chronic carriers of the hepatitis B virus with hepatitis B surface antigen (HBsAg) persisting for longer than 6 months. Chronic carriage is more frequent in those infected as children and rises to 90% in those infected perinatally.

16.1.4   Among carriers of the virus, those in whom hepatitis B e-antigen (HBeAg) is detectable are most infectious. Those with antibody to HBeAg (anti-HBe) are generally of low infectivity although a small subgroup with detectable HBV DNA are considered to be of medium infectivity.

16.1.5   A proportion of antigen carriers develop chronic hepatitis. Sometimes there is impairment of liver function tests; biopsy findings range from normal to active hepatitis, with or without cirrhosis. The prognosis of the liver disease in such individuals is at present uncertain, but it is known that some will develop hepatocellular carcinoma.

16.1.6   The number of overt cases of hepatitis B in the UK is low and there has been a marked decrease in recent years. Notifications of acute hepatitis B to the Public Health Laboratory Service fell from a peak of just under 2000 reports from England in 1984 to just over 500 reports in 1990.

Figure 16.1 shows reports to PHLS of acute hepatitis B from 1975 to 1990.

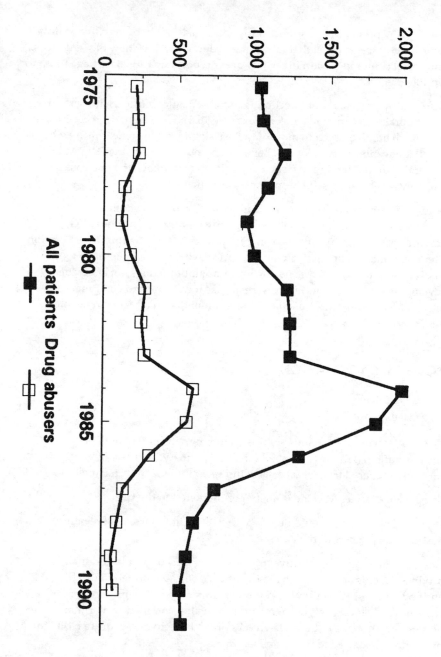

Figure 16.1   Acute hepatitis B PHLS reports

All patients Drug abusers

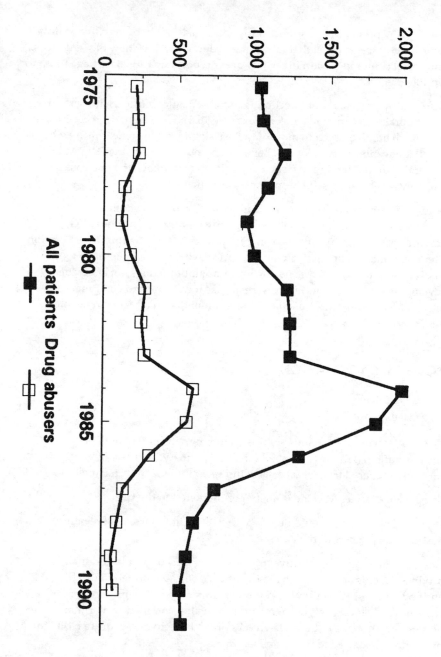

Hepatitis B

16.1.7   The prevalence of surface antigenaemia is not known with certainty but recent figures suggest that it is in the order of 1 in 1500 new blood donors. Ante-natal clinics in certain inner-city areas report hepatitis B carriage in up to 1 in 100 women.

16.1.8   The prevalence of infection is increased among those with certain behavioural or occupational risk factors (see 16.4). The recent decrease in acute hepatitis B has been seen in most of these risk groups. In some, this may be linked to the modification of risk behaviours in response to the HIV/AIDS epidemic but in other groups, such as health care workers, the decrease probably reflects successful immunisation policy.

16.1.9   There are two types of immunisation product; a vaccine which produces an immune response, and a specific immunoglobulin (HBIG) which provides passive immunity and can give immediate but temporary protection after accidental inoculation or contamination with antigen positive blood. Passive immunisation with specific immunoglobulin does not affect the development of active immunity in response to vaccine and combined active/passive immunisation may be recommended in certain circumstances (see 16.11).

ACTIVE IMMUNISATION

16.2   Vaccine

16.2.1   Hepatitis B vaccine contains 20 micrograms per ml of hepatitis B surface antigen (HBsAg) adsorbed on aluminium hydroxide adjuvant. It is currently prepared from yeast cells using recombinant DNA technology.

The plasma-derived vaccine is no longer marketed in the UK.

16.2.2   The vaccine should be stored at 2–8°C but not frozen. **Freezing destroys the potency of the vaccine.**

16.2.3   The vaccine is effective in preventing infection in individuals who produce specific antibodies to the hepatitis B surface antigen (anti-HBs). An antibody level of 100 miu/ml is generally considered to be protective. Those with antibody levels below 100 miu/ml soon after completing a primary course of immunisation may not be effectively protected and may require HBIG for protection if exposed to infection (see 16.11).

Overall, about 80-90% of individuals mount a response to the vaccine. Those over the age of 40 are less likely to respond. Patients who are immunodeficient or on immunosuppressive therapy may respond less well than healthy individuals and may require larger doses of vaccine or an additional dose.

Immunisation may take up to six months to confer adequate protection when the usual dosage schedule is followed (see 16.5.1).

Antibody titres should be checked two to four months after its completion. Poor responders (anti-HBs 10-100 miu/ml) and non-responders (anti-HBs ‹10 miu/ml) should be considered for a booster dose or, possibly, for a repeat course of vaccine.

The duration of antibody persistence is not known precisely. At present it is considered that individuals who continue to be at risk of infection should receive a booster dose three to five years after the primary course unless they have already received a booster dose following possible exposure to the virus (see 16.11.2).

Antibody levels greater than 100 miu/ml persist in some individuals for much longer than 5 years and there is some evidence that protective immunity is still present when antibody levels have fallen below 100 miu/ml.

16.3 Recommendations

16.3.1   Immunisation is recommended in individuals who are at increased risk of hepatitis B because of their occupation, lifestyle or other factors such as close contact with a case or carrier. In some groups the risk is similar for all but, in other cases, it will be necessary for an individual assessment of risk to be made. This is particularly the case with those who may be at risk because of their occupation.

NB. It is important that immunisation against hepatitis B does not encourage relaxation of good infection-control procedures.

16.3.2   The vaccine should **not** be given to individuals known to be hepatitis B surface antigen positive, or to patients with acute hepatitis B, since in the former case it would be unnecessary and, in the latter, ineffective.

Hepatitis B vaccine **may** be given to HIV positive individuals.

16.3.3   Screening for hepatitis B markers prior to immunisation may sometimes be considered in a population where the antibody prevalence is expected to be high and will also depend on the local cost and availability of screening tests.

16.4 Risk groups

16.4.1   Parenteral drug abusers.

16.4.2   Individuals who frequently change sexual partners, particularly homosexual and bisexual men and prostitute men and women.

16.4.3   Close family contacts of a case or carrier.

Sexual partners are most at risk but close household contacts may also be at increased risk.

Contacts should be checked to see if they have already been infected. Contacts who are HBsAg, anti-HBs or anti-HBc positive do not require immunisation but, in the case of sexual partners, it may be unwise to delay administration of the first dose of vaccine whilst awaiting test results. Advice regarding the use of condoms until immunity is established should be considered.

Sexual contacts of patients with acute hepatitis B should also receive HBIG (see 16.11).

16.4.4   Babies born to mothers who are chronic carriers of the hepatitis B virus or who have had acute hepatitis B during pregnancy.

Recent studies have shown that selective screening of ante-natal patients fails to identify some carriers. This is due not only to a failure to correctly identify those with established risk factors but also to the existence of some carriers who have no obvious risk factors for hepatitis B. Ante-natal clinics should therefore consider offering screening to all ante-natal patients for HBsAg and, if positive, for e-antigen status. Some clinics already do so.

Babies born to mothers who are HBeAg positive, who are HBsAg positive without e markers or who have had acute hepatitis B during pregnancy should receive HBIG as well as active immunisation (see 16.11).

16.4.5   Haemophiliacs, those receiving regular blood transfusions or blood products, or relatives responsible for the administration of such products.

16.4.6   Patients with chronic renal failure. The response to hepatitis B vaccine is poor in those who are immunocompromised. Only about 60% of patients on haemodialysis develop anti-HBs and therefore the early immunisation of those with chronic renal failure is recommended.

16.4.7   Health care personnel who have direct contact with blood or blood-stained body fluids or with patients' tissues.

This group will include doctors, surgeons, dentists, nurses, midwives, laboratory workers and mortuary technicians but immunisation should also be considered for other staff who are at risk of injury from blood-stained sharp instruments, contamination of surface lesions by blood or blood-stained body fluids or of being deliberately injured or bitten by patients.

16.4.8   Trainee health care workers.

16.4.9   Other occupational risk groups.

In some occupational groups, such as morticians and embalmers, there is an established risk of hepatitis B. In other groups, the incidence of infection is not apparently greater than in the population as a whole. This applies to members of the police, ambulance, rescue services and staff of custodial institutions. Nevertheless, there may be individuals within these occupations who are at higher risk and who should be considered for immunisation. Such a selection has to be decided locally by the occupational health services or as a result of appropriate medical advice.

16.4.10   Staff and clients of residential accommodation for the mentally handicapped.

A higher prevalence of hepatitis B carriage has been found among certain groups of the mentally handicapped in residential accommodation than in the general population. Close daily living contact and the possibility of behavioural problems may lead to staff and other clients being at increased risk of infection.

16.4.11   Inmates of custodial institutions, who will be in custody for at least 6 months and those in custody for shorter periods who belong to other risk groups.

16.4.12   Those travelling to areas of high prevalence who intend to seek employment as health care workers or who plan to remain there for lengthy periods and who may therefore be at increased risk of acquiring infection as the result of medical or dental procedures carried out in those countries.

Short term tourists or business travellers are not generally at increased risk of infection but they may place themselves at risk by their sexual behaviour when abroad.

16.5   Route of administration and dosage

16.5.1   The basic immunisation regimen consists of three doses of vaccine, with the first dose at the elected date, the second dose one month later and the third dose at six months after the first dose.

An accelerated schedule has also been used where more rapid immunisation is required, for example with travellers or following exposure to the virus, when the third dose may be given at two months after the initial dose with a booster dose at 12 months.

The vaccine should normally be given intramuscularly. The injection should be given in the deltoid region, though the anterolateral thigh is the preferred site for infants. The buttock must not be used because vaccine efficacy may be reduced.

In patients with haemophilia, the intradermal or subcutaneous route may be used. The likelihood of an effective antibody response is, however, reduced following use of the intradermal route and doctors are advised that until such time as the manufacturers apply for and are granted variations to their product licences for the intradermal route of administration, the use of this route is on their own personal responsibility.

16.5.2 **Dosage**

Age 0–12 years   10 mcg (0.5 ml)
Adults   20 mcg (1.0 ml)

The intradermal dose (but see 16.5.1) is 2 micrograms (0.1 ml).

16.6   Adverse reactions

Hepatitis B vaccine is generally well tolerated and the most common adverse reactions are soreness and redness at the injection site. Injection intradermally may produce a persisting nodule at the site of the injection, sometimes with local pigmentation changes. Other reactions which have been reported include fever, rash, malaise and an influenza-like syndrome, arthritis, arthralgia, myalgia and abnormal liver function tests.

It is important that adverse reactions should be reported to the Committee on Safety of Medicines by the yellow card system.

16.7   Contraindications

Immunisation should be postponed in individuals suffering from severe febrile infections.

16.8   Pregnancy

Hepatitis B infection in pregnant women may result in severe disease for the mother and chronic infection of the newborn. Immunisation should not be withheld from a pregnant woman if she is in a high risk category.

Information available on the outcome in those immunised during pregnancy does not reveal any cause for concern.

16.9   Supplies of Hepatitis B Vaccine

Engerix B   SmithKline Beecham. Tel. 0707 325111

16.10   Post-exposure prophylaxis

16.10.1   Specific hepatitis B immunoglobulin (HBIG) is available for passive protection and is normally used in combination with hepatitis B vaccine to confer passive/active immunity after exposure.

16.10.2   Whenever immediate protection is required, immunisation with the vaccine should be combined with simultaneous administration of hepatitis B immunoglobulin (HBIG) at a different site. It has been shown that passive immunisation with HBIG does not suppress an active immune response. A single dose of HBIG (usually 500 Iu for adults; 200 Iu for the newborn) is sufficient for healthy individuals. If infection has already occurred at the time of immunisation, virus multiplication may not be inhibited completely, but severe illness and, most importantly, the development of the carrier state may be prevented.

16.10.3   Immunoglobulin should be administered as soon as possible after exposure. In babies exposed at birth it should be given no later than 48 hours after birth (but see 16.11.1) and in other types of exposure it should preferably be given within 48 hours and certainly no later than a week after exposure.

16.10.4   There is no evidence associating the administration of HBIG with acquisition of HIV infection. Not only does the processing of the plasma from which it is prepared render it safe, but the screening of blood donations is now routine practice.

16.11   Groups requiring post-exposure prophylaxis

16.11.1   Babies born to mothers who are HBeAg positive carriers, who are HBsAg positive without e markers or who have had acute hepatitis B during pregnancy.

Active/passive immunisation is recommended (see 16.4.4). The first dose of vaccine should be given at birth or as soon as possible thereafter. HBIG should be given at a contralateral site at the same time; arrangements should be made well in advance. If administration of HBIG is delayed for more than 48 hours, advice should be sought from the local Consultant in Communicable Disease Control, a Consultant in Medical Microbiology or from the PHLS Communicable Diseases Surveillance Centre.

16.11.2   Persons who are accidentally inoculated, or who contaminate the eye or mouth or fresh cuts or abrasions of the skin, with blood from a known HBsAg positive person. Individuals who sustain such accidents should wash the affected area well with soap and warm water and seek medical advice. Advice about prophylaxis after such accidents should be obtained by telephone from the nearest Public Health Laboratory. Advice following accidental exposure may also be obtained from the Hospital Control of Infection Officer or the Occupational Health Services.

Health care workers who have already been successfully immunised should be given a booster dose of vaccine unless they are known to have adequate protective levels of antibody.

Guidance on the management of inoculation injuries from sources for which the hepatitis B status is unknown is contained in "Guidance for Clinical Health Care Workers: Protection against Infection with HIV and Hepatitis Viruses" (HMSO 1990).

16.11.3   Sexual consorts (and in some circumstances a family contact judged to be at high risk) of individuals suffering from acute hepatitis B, and who are seen within one week of onset of jaundice in the contact.

16.12   Dosage

Hepatitis B immunoglobulin is available in 2ml ampoules containing 200 Iu and 5ml ampoules containing 500 Iu.

> *Newborn*   200 Iu as soon as possible after birth.

> If administration of HBIG is delayed for more than 48 hours see 16.11.1.

> *Children*
> | Age 0–4 years | 200 Iu |
> | Age 5–9 years | 300 Iu |

> *Adults and children aged 10 years or more*   500 Iu

> For adults and children not exposed at birth, HBIG should be given preferably within 48 hours and not later than a week after exposure.

16.13   Supplies of Hepatitis B Immunoglobulin

Public Health Laboratory Service: either from the Communicable Disease Surveillance Centre (Tel. 081-200 6868) or via local Public Health Laboratories.

In Scotland, Hepatitis B immunoglobulin is held by the Blood Transfusion Service:

Aberdeen	(0224) 681818
Dundee	(0382) 645166
Edinburgh	(031) 2297291
Glasgow	(0698) 373315/8

Inverness   (0463) 234151

In Northern Ireland, Hepatitis B immunoglobulin is held by the Regional Virus Laboratory, Royal Victoria Hospital, Belfast. Tel (0232) 240503.

Note: Supplies of this product are limited and demands should be restricted to patients in whom there is a clear indication for its use.

Hepatitis B

17 Immunisation for Foreign Travel

17.1 Introduction

17.1.1 Health advice for travellers is becoming increasingly complex as more people travel to more remote parts of the world and new, and sometimes, unfamiliar vaccines have to be considered. This chapter summarises those vaccines to be considered for foreign travel. Full details are contained in the individual chapters.

17.1.2 Advice to an individual traveller will depend on not only the country or countries to be visited, but also the area, the season, the type of holiday, the length of stay and the age and previous health of the traveller. It must also take into account entry regulations for each country if travelling to more than one, and must allow for last minute excursions.

17.1.3 It is also important to remember that the commonest illnesses acquired abroad are preventable by measures other than vaccines:

a **Diarrhoea** occurs in up to 50% of travellers abroad. It and other diseases related to poor hygiene and sanitation such as hepatitis A and typhoid, is largely preventable by keeping to simple rules regarding personal hygiene and the food and drink consumed.

b **Malaria** – about 2000 cases of malaria are reported in the UK each year in travellers. Most are due to failure to take, or poor compliance with, malarial chemoprophylaxis.

17.2 Vaccines

See table for summary of vaccines, doses and intervals.

17.3 Recommendations

17.3.1
a **For all travellers**

This is an ideal opportunity to check that adults have completed tetanus and polio immunisations and that childhood immunisations are up-to-date.

b **For areas where there is still indigenous poliomyelitis, such as Africa, Asia and Eastern Europe**

Poliomyelitis vaccine

c   For areas of poor hygiene

Typhoid
Hepatitis A

d   For some countries, as a condition of entry

Yellow fever
Meningococcal meningitis

e   For visits to infected areas of a country

Yellow fever
Meningococcal meningitis

f   For infected areas, in some circumstances

Cholera – to satisfy unofficial border demands

Rabies – remote travel out of reach of medical attention

Japanese encephalitis – stays of more than one month in rural areas in the months during and after rainfall, usually June–September.

Tick-borne encephalitis – camping/walking in warm forested areas of North Europe in late spring–summer.

BCG – stays over one month; close contact with local population

17.3.2   Whenever possible, the recommended intervals between doses and between vaccines should be followed. Most travellers' needs can be accommodated in two visits four to six weeks apart:

First Visit

Yellow fever
Typhoid – 1st dose
Tetanus – booster
Hepatitis A – 1st dose if vaccine indicated (see 17.3.3 below)

Second Visit

Typhoid – 2nd dose
Polio – booster
Meningitis
Hepatitis A immunoglobulin – (or 2nd dose of vaccine – see note 17.3.3)

17.3.3   For short-term travel and single holiday trips, one dose of immunoglobulin gives adequate protection against hepatitis A. Hepatitis A vaccine is an alternative for those who need longer term protection or who travel frequently to endemic areas.

Immunisation for Foreign Travel

17.3.4 Where there is less than three weeks before departure, yellow fever and polio should be given on the same day.

17.3.5 If the polio and tetanus doses are the first, rather than boosters, the courses should be started earlier. If time does not allow this, the 2nd and 3rd doses can be completed after travel.

17.3.6 If rabies and/or Japanese encephalitis vaccines are required, at least one additional visit will be required.

17.3.7 For most vaccines, if time is short, a single dose will afford some useful protection.

17.4   Bibliography

1. International Travel and health
   Vaccination Requirements and Health Advice
   WHO Geneva
   Published every year

2. A guide on safe food for travellers
   WHO, 1211 Geneva 27, Switzerland
   Sf20 for 50 copies

Useful telephone numbers

CDSC Travel Unit (for enquiries from the medical profession)
Tel. 081-200 6868

Malaria Reference Laboratory
Pre-recorded message: 071 636 7921
(Egypt, Morocco, Turkey) 071 637 0248

For professional advice
9.00-10.30am and 2.00-3.00pm
071 636 3924

Hospital for Tropical Diseases Travel Clinic (for enquiries from the medical profession) Tel. 071-637 9899.

	Primary Course	Interval between doses	Reinforcing doses	Comments
Diphtheria				
< 10 years	3 doses usually as DTP	4 weeks	On exposure to a case	
> 10 years	Low dose vaccine 3 doses of 0.5ml sc or im	4 weeks		
Tetanus				
< 10 years	3 doses usually as DTP 0.5ml sc or im	4 weeks	1. At school entry or 3 years after last dose 2. Before leaving school.	
> 10 years	3 doses adsorbed vaccine of 0.5ml im or sc	4 weeks	1. 10 years after primary course 2. 10 years later.	
Poliomyelitis				
OPV	3 doses	4 weeks	1. At school entry. 2. Before leaving school. 3. Every 10 years if at continuing risk.	Faecal excretion of vaccine virus up to 6/52; may be longer in immune suppressed.
IPV	3 doses 0.5ml sc or im	4 weeks	As above.	

Continued

Immunisation for Foreign Travel

	Primary Course	Interval between doses	Reinforcing doses	Comments
Hepatitis A				
(vaccine adults (only)	2 doses 1.0ml im	2–4 weeks	Single booster 6–12 months after primary course	
Immunoglobulin < 10 years	2/12 protection: 125 mg	3–5/12 protection 250 mg im		
> 10 years	2/12 protection: 250 mg	3–5/12 protection 500 mg im		
Typhoid Heat killed phenol preserved				
> 10	0.5ml sc or im then 0.5ml sc or im or 0.1ml id	4–6 weeks Valid > 10 days	0.5ml im or sc or 0.1ml id every 3 years	
1–10 Vi antigen	0.25ml sc or im then 0.25 ml sc or im or 0.1ml id		0.25ml im or sc or 0.1ml id every 3 years or as required for travel	
Cholera > 10 years	1 dose 0.5ml sc or im		1.0ml)	
1–10 years	0.3ml sc or im		0.5ml)	
1–5 years	0.1 mc or im		0.3ml) every 6 months or as required for travel	
Yellow fever > 9/12	1 dose 0.5ml sc		Every 10 years	Given at designated centres only

	Primary Course	Interval between doses	Reinforcing doses	Comments
Meningococcal A + C				
> 2/12	1 dose 0.5ml sc or im		Every 3 years	May be less effective < 2 years of age
Rabies				
> 1 year	3 doses 1.0ml sc or im or 0.1m 1 id (but see text)	0, 7 and 28 days	Every 2–3 years	
Japanese Encephalitis				
children < 3 years half dose	3 doses 1.0ml sc	0, 7–14 and 28 days	> 3 years × 1	Unlicensed named patient only
	2 doses 1.0ml sc	4 weeks	> 1 year × 1	Gives immunity for 1 year
Tick Borne Encephalitis				
	3 doses 0.5ml im	0, 4–12 weeks then 9–12 months	Single dose × 1 up to 6 years > 10 course	Unlicensed vaccine – named patients only
	2 doses 0.5ml im	4–12 weeks	Protection 1 year	
BCG				
	1 (> Heaf testing) 0.1ml id		None	Valid after 2 months

Immunisation for Foreign Travel

18   Rabies

18.1   Introduction

18.1.1   Rabies is an acute viral infection resulting in encephalomyelitis. The onset is insidious. Early symptoms may include paraesthesiae around the site of the wound, fever, headache and malaise. The disease may present in one of three ways: spasms, or hydrophobia, hallucinations, and maniacal behaviour progressing to paralysis and coma, or an ascending flaccid paralysis and sensory disturbance. Rabies is almost always fatal, death resulting from respiratory paralysis. The incubation period is generally between two and eight weeks, but may range from nine days to two years.

18.1.2   Infection is usually via the bite of a rabid animal. Rarely, transmission of the virus can also occur through mucous membranes. It does not occur through intact skin. Person-to-person spread of the disease is extremely rare, but instances of transmission by corneal graft have been reported. No case of indigenous human rabies has been reported in the United Kingdom since 1902 although cases occur in persons infected abroad. The disease occurs in all continents except Australasia and Antarctica. Rabies in animals has spread throughout a great part of Central and Western Europe since 1945 and continues to advance westwards. In Europe foxes are predominantly infected but many other animals become infected including dogs and cats, cattle, horses, badgers, martens and deer. In the United States, rabies in animals has become more prevalent since the 1950's; skunks, raccoons and bats account for 85% of animal cases.

18.2   Vaccine

18.2.1   Rabies vaccine is used for pre-exposure protection of individuals at high risk and, with rabies specific immunoglobulin if necessary, for rabies post-exposure treatment. Human diploid cell rabies vaccine (HDCV) is a freeze dried suspension of Wistar rabies virus strain PM/WI 38 1503-3M cultured on human diploid cells and inactivated by beta-propiolactone. The potency of the reconstituted vaccine is not less than 2.5 International Units per 1ml dose. The freeze dried vaccine should be stored at 2–8°C and not frozen. It should be used immediately after reconstitution with the diluent supplied and any unused vaccine discarded after one hour. It may be given by deep subcutaneous, intramuscular or intradermal injection, usually into the deltoid region. The vaccine contains traces of neomycin.

18.2.2   Rabies-specific immunoglobulin

Human rabies immunoglobulin (HRIG) is obtained from the plasma of immunised human donors. It is used after exposure to rabies to give rapid protection until rabies vaccine, which should be given at the same time, becomes effective. Up to half the calculated dose is infiltrated in and around the wound after thorough cleansing, and the rest is given by intra-muscular injection into the gluteal region.

18.3   Recommendations

18.3.1   Pre-exposure prophylaxis

Pre-exposure immunisation should be offered to those in the following categories:

a   Laboratory workers handling the virus.

b   Those, who by the nature of their work, are likely to have contact with imported animals eg.

- at animal quarantine centres
- at zoos,
- at research and acclimatisation centres where primates and other imported animals are housed
- at ports eg. Customs and Excise officers
- carrying agents authorised to carry imported animals
- veterinary and technical staff at the Ministry of Agriculture, Fisheries and Food (MAFF) and Department of Agriculture and Fisheries for Scotland (DAFS).
- inspectors appointed by local authorities under the Diseases of Animals Act.

c   Workers in enzootic areas abroad who by the nature of their work are at special risk (eg. veterinary staff or zoologists).

d   Health workers who come into close contact with a patient with rabies.

e   Those living or travelling in enzootic areas who may be exposed to unusual risk of being infected or are undertaking especially long journeys in remote parts where medical treatment may not be immediately available.

Rabies vaccine is free from the NHS for those at **occupational** risk at home and abroad, ie. those in categories (**a**)–(**d**) above, but not for those in category (**e**).

18.3.2   For primary pre-exposure protection, three 1.0ml doses of HDVC should be given, one each on days 0, 7 and 28, by deep subcutaneous or intramuscular injection in the deltoid region. (The antibody response may be reduced if the gluteal region is used.) All travellers to enzootic areas should also be informed by their medical advisers of the practical steps to be taken if an animal bite is sustained (see 18.3.4).

18.3.3 **Use of the intradermal route:** When more than one person is to be immunised, the vaccine may be administered in smaller doses (0.1ml) by the intradermal route with the same time intervals as above. The intradermal route may also be used for rapid immunisation of, for example, staff caring for a patient with rabies, giving 0.1ml of vaccine intradermally into each limb (0.4ml in all) on the first day of exposure to the patient. **Intradermal immunisation is reliable only if the whole of the 0.1ml dose is properly given into the dermis and should only be given by those experienced in the intradermal technique. It should not be used in those taking chloroquine for malaria prophylaxis as this suppresses the antibody response. The use of the intradermal route is on the doctor's own responsibility as this is not covered by the manufacturer's Product Licence.**

18.3.4 Single reinforcing doses of vaccine should be given at two to three year intervals to those at continued risk.

18.3.5 The three dose primary pre-exposure course produces protective antibody in virtually 100% of recipients and makes routine post-immunisation serological testing unnecessary. Serological testing is advised for those who work with live virus. They should have their antibodies tested every six months, and be given reinforcing doses of vaccine as necessary to maintain protective levels. Serological testing is otherwise only advised for those who have had a severe reaction to a previous dose of vaccine to confirm the necessity of a reinforcing dose.

18.3.6 **Post exposure treatment**

In the event of possible exposure, firstly, as soon as possible after the incident, the wound should be thoroughly cleansed by scrubbing with soap and water under a running tap for five minutes. Secondly, the name and address of the owner of the animal should be obtained and the animal observed for ten days to see if it begins to behave abnormally. If necessary, the assistance of local officials should be sought. Thirdly, advice should be taken from a local doctor. If the animal is wild or a stray and observation is impossible, the doctor will know if rabies occurs in the locality and if immunisation is advised.

18.3.7 For travellers returning to this country who report an exposure to an animal abroad, treatment, including cleaning the wound as above, should be started as soon as possible while enquiries are made about the prevalence of rabies in the country concerned, and where possible, the ownership and condition of the biting animal. Information should be sought from the PHLS Virus Reference Division, PHLS, London (081-200 4400); in Scotland, the

Communicable Diseases (Scotland) Unit (041-946 7120); in Northern Ireland, DHSS (0232 650111).

18.3.8   Previously unimmunised individuals should be given:

a   1.0ml of HDCV by deep subcutaneous or intramuscular injection followed by five further doses on days 3, 7, 14, 30 and 90. (The day of the first dose is day 0.) The vaccine should be given into the deltoid region, or in a child, the anterolateral aspect of the thigh.

b   rabies specific immunoglobulin, 20iu/kg body weight. Up to half the dose is infiltrated in and around the wound after cleansing and the rest given by intramuscular injection.

The treatment schedule may be stopped if the animal concerned is found conclusively to be free of rabies.

18.3.9   Previously fully immunised individuals should be given two doses of HDCV 1.0ml intramuscularly into the deltoid (not buttock) on days 0 and 3-7.

Immunoglobulin treatment is not needed.

Advice should be obtained from the Virus Reference Division, Central Public Health Laboratory, Colindale, London (081-200 4400).

18.3.10   WHO recommendations for treatment are given in the WHO Expert Committee Report (see 18.7).

18.3.11   Human rabies is a notifiable disease. In the event of a case of human rabies, the Consultant in Communicable Disease Control (in Scotland the Chief Administrative Medical Officer) should be informed.

18.4   Adverse reactions

18.4.1   HDCV may cause local reactions such as redness, swelling or pain at the site of injection within 24–48 hours of administration. Systemic reactions such as headache, fever, muscle aches, vomiting, and urticarial rashes have been reported. Anaphylactic shock has been reported from the USA and Guillain-Barré syndrome from Norway. Reactions may become more severe with repeated doses.

18.4.2   HRIG may cause local pain and low grade fever but no serious adverse reactions have been reported.

18.4.3   Suspected adverse reactions should be reported to the Committee on Safety of Medicines using the yellow card system.

Rabies

18.5 Contraindications

18.5.1   There are no absolute contraindications to HDCV, although if there were evidence of hypersensitivity, subsequent doses should not be given except for treatment.

18.5.2   Pre-exposure vaccine should only be given to pregnant women if the risk of exposure to rabies is high.

18.6 Supplies

18.6.1   Human diploid cell vaccine (HDCV) is manufactured by Institut Merieux, France, and is available from Merieux UK (Tel 0628 785291).

HDCV for those at occupational risk is supplied by DH and is available from the PHLS Virus Reference Division, Tel. 081-200 4400. For persons not in categories (a)–(d) in paragraph 18.3.1 vaccine is not available on NHS prescription. It can be obtained through local pharmacies by private prescription.

For post-exposure use, vaccine is supplied by centres listed in the PHLS Directory. Information may be obtained from PHLS Virus Reference Division, CD Scotland Unit, or DHSS Northern Ireland (see 18.3.7).

18.6.2   Human rabies immunoglobulin (HRIG) is manufactured by Bio Products Laboratory (BPL) and supplied through some Public Health Laboratories (see above), also BPL and the SNBTS.

Supply centres in Scotland for HDVC and HRIG are listed in the SHID Memorandum on Rabies. In Ireland, HRIG is available from The Laboratories, Belfast City Hospital (Tel. 0232 329241).

18.7 Bibliography

WHO Expert Committee on Rabies, 7th report
Technical Report Services, 709 WHO Geneva 1984.

19   Cholera

19.1   Introduction

19.1.1   Cholera is an acute diarrhoeal illness caused by an enterotoxin produced by *Vibrio cholera* which have colonised the small bowel. The illness is characterised by the sudden onset of profuse, watery stools with occasional vomiting. Dehydration, metabolic acidosis and circulatory collapse may follow rapidly. Untreated, over 50% of the most severe cases die within a few hours of onset; with prompt, correct treatment, mortality is less than 1%. Mild cases with only moderate diarrhoea also occur and asymptomatic infection is common. The incubation period is usually between two and five days but may be only a few hours.

19.1.2   The disease is mainly water-borne, infection being acquired by the ingestion of contaminated water, shellfish or other food. However, even in infected areas the risk to travellers is very small.

19.1.3   Cholera due to the classical biotype of V. cholera was endemic in the Ganges Delta of West Bengal and Bangladesh during the last two centuries and caused epidemics and global pandemics. The seventh global pandemic which started in 1961 is due to the El Tor biotype. Cholera is now widespread in the Far East, Africa and South America.

19.1.4   The last indigenous case of cholera in England and Wales was reported in 1893. Occasional imported cases occur, but the risk of an outbreak is very small in countries with modern sanitation and water supplies and high standards of food hygiene.

19.1.5   Prevention of cholera depends primarily on improving sanitation and water supplies in endemic areas and on scrupulous personal and food and water hygiene. Cholera vaccine gives only limited personal protection and does not prevent spread of the disease. The World Health Organisation (WHO) therefore no longer recommends use of the vaccine, and immunisation against cholera is no longer a legal requirement for entry into any foreign country.

19.2   Vaccine

19.2.1   Cholera vaccine contains a mixture of the heat-killed, phenol-preserved Inaba and Ogawa serotypes of vibrio cholera at a concentration of not less than 8,000 million organisms/ml. It gives at the most 50% protection against both the classical and El Tor biotypes. The protection conferred lasts only three to six months and is minimal one year after the last dose.

19.2.2   The vaccine should be stored at 2–8°C. It has a tendency, on standing, to settle out in a gelatinous form. Vigorous shaking will yield a homogeneous suspension suitable for injection. Any partly used multi-dose containers should be discarded at the end of the immunisation session.

19.3   Recommendations

19.3.1   Cholera vaccine should not be required of any traveller. However, border officials acting unofficially may sometimes ask people travelling from infected areas for evidence of immunisation. Travellers who are likely to cross borders from such areas, especially overland, should therefore be advised to have the vaccine here before travel rather than risk having to have injections abroad.

19.3.2   Cholera vaccine is **not** indicated in the control of outbreaks or in the management of contacts of imported cases.

19.3.3   Primary immunisation consists of two doses of vaccine, given by deep subcutaneous or intramuscular injection at least one week and preferably one month apart. Booster doses are required if more than six months have elapsed since the last injection. The second and subsequent doses may be given intradermally. For the purpose of providing a certificate one injection is sufficient. The certificate is valid six days after the first dose, or immediately after a booster, and for six months.

19.3.4   **Dose**

Age	First dose	All subsequent doses	
	im or sc	im or sc	id
<1 year		not recommended	
1–5 years	0.1ml	0.3ml	0.1ml
5–10 years	0.3ml	0.5ml	0.1ml
>10 years	0.5ml	1.0ml	0.2ml

19.3.5   Cholera vaccine **may** be given to HIV positive individuals.

19.4   Adverse reactions

19.4.1   Occasional local tenderness and redness occurs at the injection site lasting one to two days, which may be accompanied by fever, malaise and headache. Serious reactions are rare.

19.4.2   Repeated immunisation may lead to hypersensitivity.

19.4.3   Serious reactions should be reported to the Committee on Safety of Medicines using the yellow card system.

19.5   Contraindications

a   Acute febrile illness

b   Hypersensitivity or other severe reaction to a previous dose.

c   Pregnancy: Although there is no information to suggest that cholera vaccine is unsafe during pregnancy it should only be given when this is unavoidable.

19.6   Managements of outbreaks

19.6.1   Cholera vaccine has **no role** in the management of contacts of any cases, or in controlling the spread of infection. Suspected cases should be notified to the CCDC or CAMO immediately. Sources of infection should be identified and treated appropriately. Contacts should maintain high standards of personal hygiene to avoid becoming infected. Control of the disease depends on public health measures rather than immunisation.

19.7   Supplies

19.7.1   Vials of 1.5ml and 10ml are available from Evans Medical Ltd Tel (0403 41400)

19.8   Bibliography

Comparative study of reactions and serological response to cholera vaccine in a controlled field trial conducted in the USSR
Burgasov P N et al
Bull WHO 1976: 54(2): 163-170

A controlled field trial of the effectiveness of intradermal and subcutaneous administration of cholera vaccine
Philippines Cholera Committee
Bull WHO 1973; 49, 389–394

Efficacy of vaccination of family contacts of cholera cases
Sommer A, Khan M, Mosley W H
Lancet 1973; (i), 1230–1232

Cholera and typhoid immunisation for foreign travel
DH, London PL/CMO(91)12 1991

Cholera

20   Typhoid

20.1   Introduction

20.1.1   Typhoid fever is a systemic infection caused by *salmonella typhi*. Most of the nearly 2000 serotypes in the genus salmonella cause only local infection of the gastro-intestinal tract (gastro-enteritis or 'food poisoning'). S typhi, S. paratyphi A, B and C and occasionally other salmonella species may invade systemically to produce a serious illness with prolonged pyrexia and prostration. The incubation period varies from one to three weeks depending on the infecting dose. All cases of typhoid and paratyphoid excrete the organisms at some stage during their illness. About 10% of patients with typhoid fever excrete the organism for three months following the acute illness and 2-5% become permanent carriers. The likelihood of becoming a chronic carrier increases with age, especially in females.

20.1.2   Typhoid fever is acquired mainly through food or drink that has been contaminated with the excreta of a human case or carrier. It is therefore predominantly a disease of countries with poor sanitation and poor standards of personal and food hygiene. Outbreaks of infection have been caused by corned beef (Aberdeen 1964), water supplies (Zermatt 1963) and shellfish contaminated by infected water or sewage. Since 1960, notifications of typhoid fever in England and Wales have remained between 100 and 200 a year. Over 80% of those have been acquired abroad, principally in the Indian Sub-continent.

20.2   Vaccine

20.2.1   Monovalent whole cell typhoid vaccine contains not less than 1000 million heat-killed, phenol-preserved S. typhi organisms per ml. One 0.5ml injection confers around 70-80% protection which fades after one year. Two doses, four to six weeks apart, give protection for three years or more.

20.2.2   A parenteral capsular polysaccharide typhoid vaccine was introduced in the UK during 1992. Each 0.5ml dose contains 25mcg of the Vi polysaccharide antigen of S. typhi preserved with phenol. A single dose gives 70-80% protection for at least three years. **This vaccine is not live.**

20.2.3   In addition, an oral typhoid vaccine is now available. Attenuated Salmonella typhi, strain TY 21a, are contained in an enteric-coated capsule. One capsule taken on alternate days for three doses appears to produce similar efficacy to parenteral vaccines, although the length of protection in those not repeatedly or constantly exposed to S. typhi may be less. **The vaccine is unstable at normal room temperatures; this vaccine is live.**

20.2.4   The efficacy of typhoid vaccines is partly related to the size of any infecting dose encountered after immunisation. The vaccines are not 100% effective and the importance in preventing infection of scrupulous attention to personal, food and water hygiene must still be emphasised for those travelling to endemic areas.

20.2.5   Typhoid vaccines should be stored at 2-8°C and not frozen. Any partly used multidose containers should be discarded at the end of the immunisation session.

20.3   Recommendations

20.3.1   Typhoid immunisation is advised for:

a   Laboratory workers handling specimens which may contain typhoid organisms.

b   Travellers to countries in Africa, Asia, Central and South America and South East Europe, especially where hygiene might be poor.

20.3.2   Typhoid immunisation is **not** recommended for contacts of a known typhoid carrier or for controlling common-source outbreaks.

20.4   Adults

20.4.1 **Whole cell vaccine**: a primary course of two doses four to six weeks apart. A reinforcing dose every three years for those at continued or repeated risk. (A single primary injection will give short-term immunity. A reinforcing dose will then be needed after one year).

20.4.2   The first dose of the primary course must be given by intramuscular or deep subcutaneous injection for a reliable antigenic response.Subsequent doses may be given by intradermal injection, which may reduce the severity of adverse reactions.

20.4.3   **Vi polysaccharide vaccine**: a single dose by intramuscular or deep subcutaneous injection. Reimmunisation with a single dose every three years for those who remain at risk of infection.

20.4.4   **Oral Ty 21a vaccine**: one capsule on alternate days for three doses. Those taking the vaccine home must be instructed to keep the vaccine in the refrigerator between doses.

20.5   Children

20.5.1   The risk of infection in children under one year is low. Immunisation against typhoid with whole cell vaccine is not recommended in this age group.

Children under 18 months may show a suboptimal response to polysaccharide antigen vaccines. Use of this vaccine in this age group should be governed by the likely risk of exposure to infection.

20.5.2   Oral typhoid vaccine is not suitable for children under six years old.

20.6   Dose

	Primary Course		Boosters
Whole Cell vaccine			
Adults	0.5ml im or deep sc		0.5ml im or sc
then	0.5ml im or deep sc	or	0.1ml id
or	0.1ml id		every three years
	4–6 weeks later		
Children	0.25ml im or deep sc		0.25ml im or deep sc
1–10 years then	0.25ml im or deep sc	or	0.1ml id every 3 years
or	0.1ml id		
	4–6 weeks later		
< one year – not recommended			
Vi polysaccharide antigen vaccine			
Adults and	0.5ml im or deep sc		0.5ml im or deep sc
children > 18/12			every 3 years
Children < 18/12	see 16.5		
Oral Ty 21a vaccine			
Adults and	1 capsule on alternate		For residents of non-
children	days × 3 doses		endemic areas:
> 6 years			3 dose course
			annually
< 6 years – not recommended			

20.7   Parenteral typhoid vaccines do not contain live organisms and may therefore be given to HIV positive individuals in the absence of contraindications. **Oral vaccine contains live organisms and is contraindicated**.

20.8   Adverse reactions

20.8.1   Whole cell typhoid vaccine commonly produces local reactions such as redness, swelling, pain and tenderness which may persist for a few days.

Systemic reactions include malaise, nausea, headache and pyrexia. They usually resolve within 36 hours. Neurological complications have been described but are rare. Reactions are especially common after repeated injections and are often more marked in people over 35 years. They may be reduced by giving the second and subsequent injections intradermally.

20.8.2   Local reactions to Vi polysaccharide vaccine are reported to be mild and transient and systemic reactions to be less common than with whole cell vaccine.

20.8.3   Oral Ty 21a vaccine may cause transient mild nausea, vomiting, abdominal cramps, diarrhoea and urticarial rash.

20.8.4   All severe reactions should be reported to the Committee on Safety of Medicines using the yellow card system.

20.9   Contraindications

20.9.1

a   Acute febrile illness

b   Severe reaction to a previous dose of the same type of vaccine

c   Pregnancy: as with other vaccines, typhoid vaccine should only be given if a clear indication exists.

d   Oral Ty 21a vaccine should not be given to those taking sulphonamides or antibiotics, and if mefloquine is being taken for malarial chemoprophylaxis the vaccine should be taken at least 12 hours before or after. It should not be given at the same time as OPV.

e   Oral typhoid vaccine is contraindicated in those with immuno-suppression due to disease or treatment.

20.9.2   Typhoid vaccine is not recommended during an outbreak of typhoid fever in the UK. It affords no immediate protection, it may temporarily increase susceptibility to infection and, by stimulating antibody production, it makes interpretation of diagnostic serological tests more difficult.

20.10   Management of outbreaks

20.10.1   The Consultant in Communicable Disease Control (CCDC) or in Scotland, the Chief Administrative Medical Officer (CAMO) should be informed immediately whenever a patient is suspected of having typhoid fever without waiting for laboratory confirmation.

20.10.2   Early identification of the source of infection is vital in containing

Typhoid

this disease. Household contacts of cases, (that is, those exposed to faeces or vomit of a case, or to the same source), should be excluded from work if **they are involved in food handling,** until at least two, and in some cases three, negative faecal cultures have been obtained. The need for strict personal hygiene should be stressed.

20.11   Supplies

20.11.1   Whole cell typhoid vaccine is available in 1.5 ml vials from Evans Medical Ltd (Tel 0403 41400).

20.11.2   Vi polysaccharide antigen vaccine is available from Merieux UK (Tel. 0628 785291)

20.11.3   Oral Ty 21a vaccine is available from Evans Medical Ltd (Tel. 0403 41400).

20.12   Bibliography

The changing pattern of food borne disease in England and Wales
Galbraith N S , Barrett N J, Sockett P N
Pub Hlth 1987; 101: 319-328.

Intradermal versus subcutaneous immunisation with typhoid vaccine
Iwarson S, Larrson P
J Hyg, Camb 1980; 84: 11–16

Protective activity of Vi capsular polysaccharide vaccine against typhoid fever
Klugman K P Et al
Lancet 1987; ii: 1166–1169

Persistence of antibody titres three years after vaccination with Vi Polysaccharide vaccine against typhoid fever
Tacket C O, Levine M M, Robbins J B
Vaccine 1988; 6 307–8

Typhoid

21   Yellow Fever

21.1   Introduction

21.1.1   Yellow fever is an acute viral infection occurring in tropical Africa and S. America; it has never been seen in Asia. It ranges in severity from non-specific symptoms to an illness of sudden onset with fever, vomiting and prostration which may progress to haemorrhage and jaundice. In indigenous populations in endemic areas fatality is about 5%; in non-indigenous individuals and during epidemics fatality may reach 50%. Two epidemiological forms, urban and jungle, are recognised although they are clinically and aetiologically identical. Only a few outbreaks of urban yellow fever have occurred in recent years. The incubation period is two to five days.

21.1.2   Urban yellow fever is spread from infected to susceptible persons by *Aedes aegypti*, a mosquito which lives and breeds in close association with man. Jungle yellow fever is a zoonosis transmitted among non-human hosts (mainly monkeys) by forest mosquitoes which may also bite and infect humans. These may, if subsequently bitten by *Aedes aegypti* become the source of outbreaks of the urban form of the disease.

21.1.3   Preventative measures against urban yellow fever include eradication of Aedes mosquitoes, protection from mosquito bites, and immunisation. Jungle fever can only be prevented by immunisation.

21.1.4   Immunisation against yellow fever, documented by a valid International Certification of Vaccination, is compulsory for entry into some countries either for all travellers or for those arriving from infected areas. Requirements should be checked at the relevant Embassy before travel.

21.2   Vaccine

21.2.1   Yellow fever vaccine is a live attenuated freeze-dried preparation of the 17D strain of yellow fever virus. Each 0.5ml dose contains not less than 1000 mouse LD50 units. It is propagated in leucosis-free chick embryos and contains no more than 2 Iu of neomycin and 5 Iu of polymyxin per dose.

21.2.2   It should be stored at 2–8°C and protected from light. The diluent supplied for use with the vaccine should be stored below 15°C but not frozen. The vaccine should be given by deep subcutaneous injection within one hour of reconstitution. Any unused vaccine should be destroyed by incineration or by disinfection at the end of the immunisation session.

21.2.3   A single dose correctly given confers immunity in nearly 100% of recipients; immunity persists for at least ten years and may be for life.

Yellow Fever

21.2.4   Yellow fever vaccine is given only at designated centres as listed in Appendix 1 and costs are passed on to the vaccinee.

21.3   Recommendations

21.3.1   The following should be immunised:

a   Laboratory workers handling infected material.

b   Persons aged nine months and over travelling through or living in infected areas. Immunisation under nine months is not recommended but may be performed if exposure to the risk of infection cannot be avoided.

c   Travellers requiring an International Certificate of Vaccination for entry into a country.

21.3.2   The dose is 0.5ml irrespective of age. The International Certificate is valid for ten years from the tenth day after primary immunisation and immediately after re-immunisation.

21.3.3   Re-immunisation every ten years is recommended for those at risk.

21.3.4   Normal human immunoglobulin obtained in the UK is unlikely to contain antibody to the yellow fever virus; the vaccine can therefore be given at the same time as an injection of immunoglobulin for travellers abroad.

21.4   Adverse reactions

21.4.1   Severe reactions are extremely rare. 5–10% of recipients have mild headache, myalgia, low-grade fever or soreness at the injection site five to ten days after immunisation.

21.4.2   The only serious reaction following 17D tissue culture vaccine has been the rare occurrence of encephalitis in young infants, all of whom have recovered without sequelae.

21.4.3   Severe reactions should be reported to the Committee on Safety of Medicines using the yellow card system.

21.5   Contraindications

21.5.1   The usual contraindications to a live virus vaccine should be observed (see 3.2.1 ii, iii, iv, v). Yellow fever vaccine should not be given to:

a   Persons suffering from febrile illness.

b   Patients receiving high-dose corticosteroid or immuno-suppressive treatment, including radiation.

c   Patients suffering from malignant conditions such as lymphoma, leukaemia, Hodgkin's disease or other tumours of the reticulo-endothelial system, or where the immunological mechanism may be impaired as in hypogammaglobulinaemia.

d   Pregnant women, because of the theoretical risk of fetal infection. However if a pregnant woman must travel to a high-risk area, she should be immunised since the risk from yellow fever outweighs that of immunisation.

e   Persons known to be hypersensitive to neomycin or polymyxin or to have had an anaphylactic reaction to egg. A letter stating that immunisation is contraindicated on these grounds may be acceptable in some countries. Advice should be sought from the appropriate Embassy.

f   Yellow fever vaccine should not be given to either symptomatic or asymptomatic HIV positive individuals since there is as yet insufficient evidence as to the safety of its use. Travellers should be told of this uncertainty and advised not to be immunised unless there are compelling reasons (see Section 3.4.4).

If such travellers still intend to visit countries where a yellow fever certificate is required for entry, then they should obtain a letter of exemption from a medical practitioner.

21.5.2   If more than one live vaccine is required, they should either be given at the same time in different sites or with an interval of three weeks between them.

21.5.3   Infants under nine months should only be immunised if the risk of yellow fever is unavoidable as there is a very small risk of encephalitis (21.4.2).

21.6   There is no risk of transmission from imported cases since the mosquito vector does not occur in the UK.

21.7   Supplies

Manufactured and supplied in 1, 5 and 10 dose vials to designated centres only by Evans Medical Ltd Tel. Horsham (0403 41400).

21.8   Bibliography

The duration of immunity following vaccination with the 17D strain of yellow fever virus.
Fox J P, Cabral A S.
Am. J. Hyg. 1943; 37; 93-120.

Stabilised 17D yellow fever vaccine: dose response studies, clinical reactions and effects on hepatic function.
Freestone D S et al.
J. Biol Stand. 1977: 5(3), 181-6.

Neutralising and HAI antibody to yellow fever 17 years after vaccination with 17D vaccine.
Groot H, Ribeivo R B.
Bull WHO 1962; 27; 699-707.

21.9   YELLOW FEVER IMMUNISATION CENTRES: England, Wales, Scotland, Northern Ireland and Isle of Man. – see Appendix 1.

22 Meningococcal Infection

22.1 Introduction

22.1.1 Meningococcal meningitis and septicaemia are systemic infections caused by *Neisseria meningitidis*. Meningococci are gram negative diplococci which are divided into antigenetically distinct groups, the commonest of which are B, C, A, Y and W135. They are further subdivided by type and sulphonamide sensitivity.

22.1.2 Group B strains account for approximately two thirds of all isolates submitted to the Public Health Laboratory Service Meningococcal Reference Laboratory. Group C strains contribute about one third. Group A strains are rare in this country (less than 2%) but are the epidemic strains in other parts of the world.

22.1.3 Irregular upsurges of meningococcal infection occur in the United Kingdom with the previous wave in the mid 1970s. The present upsurge began in 1984 and reached its peak in 1989/90 at the same time as the last influenza epidemic. The incidence of meningococcal disease is highest in infants followed by one to five year olds, but the recent epidemic of Group B 15 P1.16 and the new B4 strain have been associated with an increased incidence in teenagers.

Figure 22.1 shows the notifications for meningococcal meningitis from 1970 to 1991.

22.1.4 The carriage rate for all meningococci in the normal population is about 10% although rates vary with age; about 25% of young adults may be carriers at any one time.

22.1.5 Meningococci are transmitted by droplet spread or direct contact from carriers or from individuals in the early stages of the illness; the probable route of invasion is via the nasopharynx. The incubation period is two to three days, and the onset of disease varies from fulminant to insidious with mild prodromal symptoms. Early symptoms and signs are usually malaise, pyrexia and vomiting. Headache, photophobia, drowsiness or confusion, joint pains and a typical haemorrhagic rash of meningococcal septicaemia may develop. Early on, the rash may be non-specific. Patients may present in coma. In young infants particularly, the onset may be insidious and the classical signs absent. The diagnosis should be suspected in the presence of vomiting, pyrexia, irritability and, if still patent, raised anterior fontanelle tension.

22.2 Vaccine

22.2.1 Meningococcal vaccine is a purified, heat stable, lyophilised extract

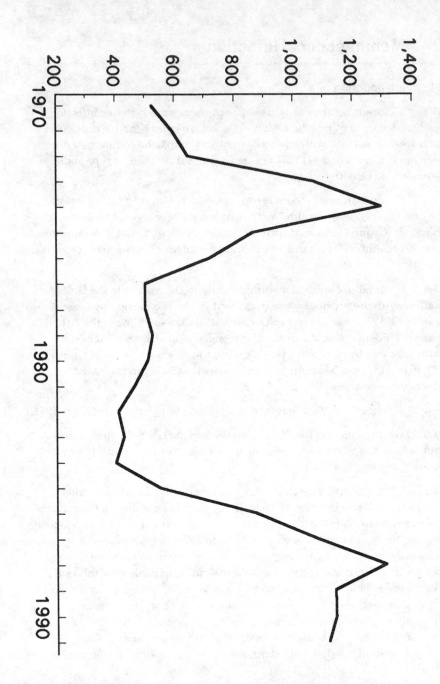

Figure 22.1 Notifications of meningococcal meningitis (E & W) 1970–1991

from the polysaccharide outer capsule of *Neisseria meningitidis*, effective against sero group A and C organisms. Vaccine contains 50mcg each of the respective purified bacterial capsular polysaccharides. **There is no available vaccine effective against Group B organisms.**

22.2.2   Vaccine must be stored at 2–8°C and the diluent must not be frozen. Vaccine should be reconstituted immediately before use with the diluent supplied by the manufacturer. A single dose of 0.5ml is given by deep subcutaneous or intramuscular injection to adults and children from two months of age.

22.2.3   A serological response is detected in more than 90% of recipients and occurs five to seven days after a single injection. The response is strictly Group specific and confers no protection against Group B organisms. Young infants respond less well than adults with little response to the Group C polysaccharide below 18 months and similar lack of response to Group A polysaccharide below three months. Vaccine induced immunity lasts approximately five years; in younger children a more rapid decline in antibody has been noted and antibodies are unlikely to persist for more than two years.

22.3   Recommendations

22.3.1   Routine immunisation with meningococcal vaccine is not recommended as the risk of meningococcal disease is very low, Group B organisms are the major cause of disease in the United Kingdom and a considerable number of cases of meningococcal disease from Group C organisms occur in children too young to be protected with presently available vaccines.

22.3.2   **Contacts of cases**: Close contacts of cases of meningococcal meningitis have a considerably increased risk of developing the disease in the subsequent months, despite appropriate chemoprophylaxis. Immediate family or close contacts of cases of Group A or Group C meningitis should be given meningococcal vaccine in addition to chemoprophylaxis. The latter should be given first and the decision to offer vaccine should be made when the results of typing are available. Vaccine should not be given to contacts of Group B cases.

22.3.3   **Local Outbreaks**: In addition to sporadic cases, outbreaks of meningococcal infections from Group C organisms tend to occur in closed or semi-closed communities such as schools and military establishments. Immunisation has been shown to be effective in controlling epidemics, reducing infection rates but not carriage rates. Advice on the use of meningococcal vaccines is available from:

Meningococcal Infection

Communicable Disease Surveillance Centre (081-200 6868).

Public Health Laboratory Service
Meningococcal Reference Laboratory (061 445 2416).

Communicable Disease (Scotland) Unit (041 946 7120).

Meningococcal Reference (Scotland) Laboratory (041 946 7120).

Meningococcal vaccine has no part to play in the management of outbreaks of Group B meningococcal meningitis.

22.3.4   **Travel**: There are areas of the world where the risk of acquiring meningococcal infection is much higher than in this country particularly for those visitors who live or travel 'rough', such as hitch-hikers or 'trekkers'. These areas include the meningitis belt of Africa where epidemics of Group A infections occur in the dry season, the area of New Delhi, Nepal and Mecca.

The meningitis belt of Africa lies mainly between latitudes 15°N and 5°N except in Uganda and Kenya where it reaches the equator.

It includes:

a   Southern Sub-Saharan parts of Senegal, Mali, Niger, Chad and Sudan.
b   All of Gambia, Guinea, Togo and Benin.
c   South-West Ethiopia.
d   Northern parts of Sierra Leone, Liberia, Ivory Coast, Nigeria, Cameroon, Central African Republic, Uganda and Kenya.

In the meningitis belt, epidemics have a seasonal character, appearing at the onset of the dry season (December–February) with a peak at the driest period when there is less than 10% relative humidity. Epidemics usually stop with the onset of the rains in May–June.

Since 1988 Saudi Arabia has required immunisation of pilgrims coming to the Haj annual pilgrimage. In 1987, there were 23 cases of Group A meningococcal meningitis in pilgrims from England or their direct contacts; in 1988 only one of 140 pilgrims returning to England carried the epidemic strain.

22.3.5   Meningococcal vaccine may be given to HIV positive individuals in the absence of contraindications.

22.4   Adverse Reactions

22.4.1   Generalised reactions are rare although pyrexia occurs more frequently in young children than in adults.

22.4.2   Injection site reactions occur in approximately 10% of recipients and last for approximately 24–48 hours.

22.4.3   Serious reactions should be reported to the Committee on Safety of Medicines using the yellow card system.

22.5   Contraindications

22.5.1   Immunisation should be postponed in individuals suffering from an acute febrile illness.

22.5.2   Although there is no information to suggest that meningococcal vaccine is unsafe during pregnancy, it should only be given when this is unavoidable, ie. required for travel. During an epidemic of meningococcal meningitis in Brazil, no adverse events were reported in pregnant women receiving vaccine.

22.5.3   A severe reaction to a preceding dose of meningococcal vaccine is a contraindication to further doses.

22.6   Supplies

22.6.1   The following meningococcal vaccines are licensed and available:

Mengivac (A+C), Merieux UK 0628 785291

ACVax, SmithKline Beecham 0707 325111

22.7   Bibliography

The epidemiology and control of meningococcal disease.
Communicable Disease Report 1989 89/08.

Antibody response to serogroup A and C polysaccharide vaccines in infants born to mothers vaccinated during pregnancy.
McCormick J B, Gusman H H et al.
J of Clin. Investigation, 1980; 65 : 1141-1144.

Meningococcus Group A vaccine in children three months to five years of age. Adverse reactions and immunogenicity related to endotoxin content and molecular weight of the polysaccharide.
Peltola H, Kayhty H, Kuronen T, Haque N, Sanna S, Makela P H.
J. Pediatr. 1978; 92 : 818-822.

Kinetics of antibody production to Group A and Group C meningococcal polysaccharide vaccines administered during the first six years of life; prospects for routine immunisation of infants and children.
Gold R, Lepow M L, Goldschneider I, Draper T F, Gotschlich E C.
J Infect dis 1979; 140 : 690-7.

Control of Meningococcal Disease.
Jones D M.
BMJ 1989; 292 : 542-543.

Secondary cases of meningococcal infection among close family and household contacts in England and Wales, 1984–7.
Cooke R P D, Riordan T, Jones D M, Painter M J.
BMJ 1989; 298: 555-558.

23 Japanese Encephalitis

23.1 Introduction

Japanese Encephalitis is a mosquito-borne viral encephalitis caused by a flavivirus antigenically related to St Louis encephalitis virus. It occurs throughout South East Asia and the Far East. Only about 1 in 200 infections becomes clinically apparent, but approximately 30% of these are fatal and a further 30% result in permanent neurological sequelae. The reservoir is infected birds and animals, and the risk of infection is greatest in rural areas, particularly where rice growing and pig farming coexist. In some countries the infection is endemic; in others the risk is greatest at the end of the rainy season (June-September).

23.2 Vaccine

A formalin-inactivated vaccine derived from mouse brain is available in the UK but is not licensed and must therefore be given on a named patient basis.

23.3 Recommendations

Immunisation is recommended only for travellers to infected areas of South East Asia and the Far East who will be staying in rural areas for more than one month. The risk to an individual traveller is difficult to assess, but areas where rice growing and pig farming coexist and journeys towards the end of the Monsoon season (June–September) are likely to increase the risk. Where individuals are likely to be at exceptional risk, vaccine could be recommended for shorter visits.

23.3.1 The recommended immunisation schedule is three doses of 1ml sc given at 0, 7-14 and 28 days. Full immunity takes up to a month to develop. A two dose schedule at 0 and 7–14 days gives protection for up to three months.

23.3.2 For children under three years of age, each injection should be 0.5ml sc.

23.3.3 A reinforcing dose should be given after one year.

23.4 Adverse reactions

i   Local reaction at the injection site may occur.

ii   Allergic reactions, mainly urticaria but also angioneurotic oedema and dyspnoea, have recently been reported from Denmark and Australia. Most reactions appear to have occurred with more recent batches.

23.4.1   Caution is therefore required with the use of this vaccine, and it is particularly important to report any suspected adverse reaction to the Committee on Safety of Medicines on a yellow card. Reports to the supplier will be passed to the Department of Health.

23.5   Contraindications

i   Fever or current active infection.

ii   Pregnancy.

iii   Cardiac, renal or hepatic disorders, leukaemia, lymphoma or other generalised malignancy.

iv   History of anaphylactic hypersensitivity.

23.6   Supplies

Biken lyophilised vaccine, produced in Japan, is available in single doses from Cambridge Selfcare Diagnostics Ltd, Tel: 091 261 5950.

24 Tick Borne Encephalitis

24.1   This disease is caused by a virus transmitted to man by the bite of an infected tick. Warm forested parts of Europe and Scandinavia, especially where there is heavy undergrowth, give the greatest risk in late spring and summer. Those walking or camping in such areas should wear clothing that covers most skin surface and use insect repellents on socks and outer clothes.

24.2   A killed vaccine is available on a named-patient basis from Immuno Limited (Telephone 0732-458101) and should be used where prolonged exposure is likely in those who work, camp or walk in the risk areas. The full primary course consists of three injections of 0.5ml (given IM), the second 4–12 weeks after the first and the third 9–12 months after the second dose. Protection then lasts three years or more and may be reinforced within a period of six years by a single dose. A shorter primary course of two injections gives protection for one year.

24.3   An immunoglobulin preparation is available from Immuno Limited, for post-exposure prophylaxis.

25 Anthrax

25.1   Anthrax is an acute bacterial disease affecting the skin and, rarely, the lungs or gastro-intestinal tract. It is caused by a spore bearing aerobic bacillus, *Bacillus anthracis* and is primarily a disease of herbivorous animals. In the UK it is rare – nine cases notified in the last ten years – and only affects workers exposed to infected hides, wool, hair, bristle, bone, bonemeal, feeding stuffs and carcasses. Spores may survive for many years, and new areas of infection may develop through the use of infected animal feed. Prevention depends on controlling anthrax in livestock and by disinfecting imported animal products. Processing of hides, wool and bone by tanning, dyeing, carbonising or acid treatment ensures that the final product carries no risk of infection. Bonemeal used as horticultural fertiliser may rarely contain anthrax spores; those handling it in bulk should wear impervious gloves which should be destroyed after use.

25.2   Vaccine

Anthrax vaccine is the alum precipitate of the antigen found in the sterile filtrate of the Sterne strain cultures of *Bacillus anthracis*, with thiomersal preservative. It must be kept at 2–8°C and should be well shaken before being given by intramuscular injection.

25.3   Recommendations

25.3.1   Immunisation against anthrax is recommended **only for workers at risk of exposure to the disease (25.1)**. Four injections of 0.5ml should be given, with intervals of three weeks between the first three injections and six months between the third and fourth. Annual reinforcing doses of 0.5ml are advised.

25.3.2   Workers at special risk should wear protective clothing. Adequate washing facilities, ventilation and dust control in hazardous industries should be provided. Prompt reporting and scrupulous medical care of skin abrasions are essential.

25.4   Adverse reactions

25.4.1   These are rare. Mild erythema and swelling lasting up to two days may occur at the site of the injection. Occasionally regional lymphadenopathy, mild fever and urticaria may develop.

25.4.2   Severe reactions should be reported to the Committee on Safety of Medicines using the yellow card system.

25.5   Contraindications

There are no specific contraindications. A local or general reaction to the first injection does not necessarily indicate a predisposition to reactions following subsequent injections.

25.6   Management of outbreaks

25.6.1   All cases of anthrax should be notified; an attempt should be made to confirm the diagnosis bacteriologically and the source of infection should be investigated. Penicillin is the treatment of choice. Skin lesions should be covered; any discharge or soiled articles should be disinfected. Anthrax vaccine has no role in the management of a case or outbreak.

25.7   Supplies

Anthrax vaccine is available from:

Public Health Laboratory Service:
Communicable Disease Surveillance Centre, Tel 081 200 6868
Centre for Applied Microbiology and Research, Tel 0980 610391
Cardiff Tel. 0222 755944
Leeds Tel. 0533 645011
Liverpool Tel. 051 525 2323

Scotland:
Perth Royal Infirmary Tel. 0738 23111
Law. Tel 0698 351100
Borders General Hospital. Tel 0896 4333

Northern Ireland:
The Laboratories, Belfast City Hospital Tel 0232 329241

25.8   Bibliography

Vaccine against anthrax.
Editorial.
BMJ 1965: ii; 717-8.

The epidemiology of anthrax.
James D G.
J Antimicrob. Chemother. 1976; 2(4); 319-20.

Thoroughly modern anthrax.
Turnbull P C.
Abstracts of Hygiene, Bureau Hyg & Trop. Dis. 1986; 61(9).

26   Smallpox and Vaccinia

26.1   In December 1979 the Global Commission for the Certification of Smallpox Eradication declared the world free of smallpox and this declaration was ratified by the World Health Assembly in May 1980.

There is thus no indication for smallpox vaccination for any individual with the exception of some laboratory staff and specific workers at identifiable risk (26.2)

26.2   Recommendations

Workers in laboratories where pox viruses (such as vaccinia) are handled, and others whose work involves an identifiable risk of exposure to pox virus, should be advised of the possible risk and vaccination should be considered. Detailed guidance for laboratory staff has been prepared by the Advisory Committee on Dangerous Pathogens and the Advisory Committee on Genetic Modification (see 26.3). Further advice on the need for vaccination and contraindications should be obtained from the Public Health Laboratory Service Virus Reference Laboratory Tel 081 200 4400; if vaccination is considered desirable, vaccine can be obtained through PHLS on this number.

26.3   Bibliography

Vaccination of laboratory workers handling vaccinia and related pox viruses infectious for humans.

Advisory Committee on Dangerous Pathogens and Advisory Committee on Genetic Modification 1990.
HMSO ISBN 0 11 885450.

Smallpox and Vaccinia

27 Varicella/Herpes Zoster

27.1 Introduction

27.1.1 Varicella (chickenpox) is an acute highly infectious disease which is transmitted directly by personal contact or droplet spread, and indirectly via fomites. In the home the secondary infection rate from a case of chickenpox can be as high as 90%. It is most common in children below the age of ten in whom it is usually mild. Vesicles appear without prodromal illness on the face and scalp, spreading to the trunk and abdomen and eventually to the limbs; after three or four days they dry with a granular scab and are usually followed by further crops. Vesicles may be so few as to be missed or so numerous that they become confluent, covering most of the body. The disease can be more serious in adults, particularly for pregnant women; for neonates and immunosuppressed individuals the risk is greatly increased (27.1.4, 27.1.5).

The incidence is seasonal and reaches a peak from March to May. The incubation period is between two and three weeks. Virus is plentiful in the naso-pharynx in the first few days and in the vesicles before they dry up; the infectious period is therefore from one to two days before the rash appears until the vesicles are dry. This may be prolonged in immunosuppressed patients.

27.1.2 Herpes zoster is caused by the reactivation of the patient's varicella virus. It is transmissible to susceptible individuals as chickenpox but there is very little evidence that it can be acquired from another individual with chickenpox. Although more common in the elderly, it can occur in children and especially in immunosuppressed individuals. Vesicles appear in the dermatome representing cranial or spinal ganglia where the virus has been dormant. The affected area may be intensely painful with associated paraesthesia.

27.1.3 Since chickenpox is so common in childhood, 90% of adults are immune. However when it occurs in adults and especially in pregnant women, it carries a risk of fulminating varicella pneumonia which can be rapidly fatal. Pregnant women with chickenpox should therefore be closely observed and admitted to hospital if necessary so that their condition can be monitored and they can be treated promptly with acyclovir.

27.1.4 Risks to the fetus and neonate from maternal chickenpox are related to the time of infection in the mother:

a In the first five months of pregnancy. Congenital varicella syndrome which includes limb hypoplasia, microcephaly, cataracts, growth retardation and skin scarring. The mortality rate is high. From a number of published studies, the incidence of congenital varicella syndrome has been estimated at 2–5% of those infected in the first four months of pregnancy. However, recent information suggests that the true risk may be below 1%.

b In the 2nd and 3rd trimesters of pregnancy. Herpes zoster in an otherwise healthy infant.

c A week before to a week after delivery. Severe and even fatal disease in the neonate. Although the risk decreases after this period it remains higher than in older children and half the deaths under one year occur during the first month of life.

27.1.5 The risk of severe or fatal varicella/zoster is increased in the following:

a Immunosuppressed individuals in whom mortality is high from disseminated infection or encephalitis.

b Individuals with debilitating disease in whom normal immunological mechanisms may be impaired.

27.2 Varicella vaccine

Liive attenuated varicella is in the process of development, but currently no vaccine is licensed for use in the UK. It is available on a named patient basis from SmithKline Beecham for immuno-compromised individuals, particularly children with leukaemia.

27.3 Human Varicella-Zoster Immunoglobulin (VZIG)

This is made in the UK by Bio Products Laboratory and distributed by the Public Health Laboratory Service (27.8). It is prepared from pooled plasma of blood donors with a history of recent chickenpox or herpes zoster, or from those who on screening are found to have suitably high titres of V-Z antibody. The V-Z antibody content of each batch is titrated and is at least eight times higher than that in normal immunoglobulin. The supply of VZIG is limited by the availability of suitable donors and its use is therefore restricted to those at greatest risk and for whom there is evidence that it is effective.

27.3.1 VZIG is a clear to pale yellow fluid supplied in ampoules containing 250 mg protein in 1.7ml of fluid with added thiomersal and sodium chloride.

27.3.2 It should be stored in a refrigerator between 2–8°C. Under these conditions it has a shelf life of three years. It can be stored for short periods at room temperature; it must **not** be frozen.

27.3.3   All immunoglobulins are prepared from HIV antibody negative donors and are treated to inactivate viruses.

27.4   Recommendations

Because of the increased risk of serious disease, VZIG is recommended for individuals in contact with chickenpox or herpes zoster in the following groups.

27.4.1   Immunosuppressed patients who within three months of the contact have been on high-dose steroids (eg. 2mg/kg/day of prednisolone for more than a week).

Wherever possible, patients in contact who are without a **definite** history of chickenpox should be screened for varicella-zoster (V-Z) antibody (27.7); only those **without** antibody require VZIG. In an emergency, antibody can be estimated within 24 hours; VZIG can be ordered (see 27.8) and returned if the test is positive.

27.4.2   Bone-marrow transplant recipients

Following contact with chickenpox or herpes zoster, these patients should be given VZIG **despite a history of chickenpox.**

NOTE: all patients on long-term immunosuppressive treatment (such as those following transplant) should be screened for V-Z antibody. Many will have antibody, among them some with a negative history of chickenpox.

27.4.3   Individuals with debilitating disease

These should be treated as in 27.4.2.

27.4.4   Infants up to four weeks after birth

VZIG is recommended for the following:

a   Those whose mothers develop chickenpox (but not zoster) in the period seven days before to one month after delivery.

b   Those in contact with chickenpox or zoster whose mothers have no history of chickenpox or who on testing have no antibody.

c   Those in contact with chickenpox who are born before 30 weeks of gestation or with a birth weight less than 1kg; these may not possess maternal antibody despite a positive history in the mother.

The following infants, aged less than one month, do not require VZIG since maternal antibody will be present:

Varicella/Zoster

d   Infants born more than seven days after the onset of maternal chickenpox.

e   Infants whose mothers have a positive history of chickenpox and/or a positive antibody result.

f   Infants whose mothers develop zoster before or after delivery.

NOTE: Neonatal varicella can still develop in infants who have received VZIG. In up to two thirds of these infants infection is mild, but rare fatal cases have occurred.

27.4.5   Pregnant women

All pregnant contacts of chickenpox without a **definite** history of chickenpox should be tested for V-Z antibody before VZIG is given since about two-thirds of women have antibody despite a negative history of chickenpox. Only those **without** antibody require VZIG.

NOTE: VZIG does not prevent infection even when given within 72 hours of exposure. However when given up to ten days after exposure it may attenuate the disease in pregnant women (27.1.4).

27.4.6   Since VZIG does not prevent infection it is not given to pregnant women with the intention of preventing congenital varicella syndrome. When supplies of VZIG are short it may not be possible to issue it for pregnant contacts of chickenpox for whom treatment with acyclovir is available.

27.5   HIV positive individuals

i)   Asymptomatic HIV positive individuals do **not** require VZIG after contact with chickenpox since there is no evidence of increased risk of serious illness in these individuals.

ii)   HIV positive individuals with symptoms should be given VZIG after contact with chickenpox unless they are known to have V-Z antibodies.

27.6   Dose of VZIG for prophylaxis

0 – 5 years	250 mg
6 – 10 years	500 mg
11 – 14 years	750 mg
15 –	1000 mg

This is given by **intramuscular** injection as soon as possible and not later than ten days after exposure. It must **not** be given intravenously.

If a second exposure occurs after three weeks, a further dose is required.

Varicella/Zoster

27.7   Treatment

There is no evidence that VZIG is effective in the treatment of severe disease. Acyclovir should be used for such cases. Since antibody production can be delayed in immunosuppressed individuals, intravenous commercial preparations of normal human immunoglobulin may be used to provide an immediate source of antibody.

27.8   Supplies

VZIG is made by Bio Products Laboratory (Tel. 081 953 6191) and distributed by all Public Health Laboratories and by Communicable Disease Surveillance Centre (CDSC) (Tel. 081 200 6868).

Northern Ireland : The Laboratories, Belfast City Hospital Tel. 0232 323241

No commercial preparation of VZIG is available.

27.9   VZIG is well tolerated. Very rarely anaphylactoid reactions occur in individuals with hypogammaglobulinaemia who have IgA antibodies, or those who have had an atypical reaction to blood transfusion

27.10   Severe reactions should be reported to the Committee on Safety of Medicines using the yellow card system.

27.11   Management of hospital outbreaks

27.11.1   Susceptible staff exposed to chickenpox should whenever possible be excluded from contact with high risk patients from eight to 21 days after exposure to a case of chickenpox or zoster.

27.11.2   To simplify procedure after the introduction of a case, it is recommended that hospital staff without a definite history of chickenpox should be routinely screened for V-Z antibody so that those susceptible are already identified. This is particularly important for staff in contact with high risk groups such as pregnant women and immunosuppressed patients.

27.12   For advice on testing for V-Z antibody, contact local Public Health or Hospital Laboratory.

Varicella/Zoster

Appendix 1

ABINGDON

Dr R Lynch-Blosse
The Surgery
Clifton Hampden
Abingdon
Oxfordshire
Tel: 0086-730 7888

Dr N R Crossley
The Abingdon Surgery
65 Street Surgery
Abingdon
Oxfordshire
OX14 3LB
Tel: 0235-523126

ADDLESTONE

Professor P R Grob
The Crouch Old Family
   Practice
45 Station Road
Addlestone
Surrey
KT15 2BH
Tel: 0932-840123/4

ALDBROUGH

Dr W J Isherwood
The Surgery
Cross Street
Aldbrough
North Humberside
HU11 4RW
0964-527497

ALDERSHOT

Dr B Robertson
North Lane Surgery
38 North Lane
Aldershot
Hampshire
GU12 4QG
Tel: 0252-344434

Dr J C Healey
Burnside Surgery
41 Connaught Road
Fleet
Aldershot
GU13 9QZ
Tel: 0252-613327

ALFORD

Dr K Charlton
Alford Group of Doctors
Merton Lodge
West Street
Alford
Lincs
LN13 9DH
Tel: 05212-3262

ALFRETON

Dr G A Richmond
The Surgery
Limes Avenue
Alfreton
Derbyshire
DE5 7DW
Tel: 0773-832525

ALTON

Dr A J Sword
Alton Health Centre
Anstey Road
Alton
GU34 2QX
Tel: 0420-84676

ALTRINCHAM

Dr M R Underwood
Group Surgery
Normans Place
Off Regent Road
Altrincham
Cheshire
WA14 2AV
Tel: 061-928 2424

Dr C Westwood
Timperley Health Centre
169 Grove Lane
Timperley
Altrincham
Cheshire
WA15 6PH
Tel: 0252-613327

AMBLESIDE

Dr I J Birket
The Health Centre
Rydall Road
Ambleside
Cumbria
Yorkshire
LA22 9BP
Tel: 0539-432693

ANDOVER

Dr T W I Lovel
Shepherds Spring Medical
   Centre
Cricketers Way
Andover
Hampshire
SP10 5DE
Tel: 0264-61126

Dr L A Davies
Charlton Hill Surgery
Charlton Road
Andover
Hampshire
SP10 3JY
Tel: 0264-337979

Dr P A Collins
Andover Health Centre
Charlton
Andover
Hants
SP10 3LD
Tel: 0264-365031

ANNESLEY WOODHOUSE

Dr G Place
194 Forest Road
Annesley Woodhouse
Nottinghamshire
NG17 9JB
Tel: 0623-752295

ASCOT

Dr P N Whitfield
King's Corner Surgery
Sunninghill
Ascot
Berkshire
SL5 OAE
Tel: 0344-23181

ASHBOURNE

Dr P R Kirtley
The Health Centre
Ashbourne
Derbyshire
DE6 1EN
Tel: 0335-300588

Dr Ian St Clair Macleod
Ashbourne Health Centre
Compton
Ashbourne
Derbyshire
DE6 1GN
Tel: 0335-43784

ASHBY DE LA ZOUCH

Dr A Bajpai
Ashby Health Centre
North Street
Ashby De La Zouch
Leicestershire
LE6 5HU
Tel: 0530-414131

ASHFORD

Dr P Kandela
The Surgery
107 Feltham Hill Road
Ashford
Middlesex
TW15 1HH
Tel: 0784-252027

Dr V S Zammit
Studholme Surgery
50 Chrch Road
Ashford
Middlesex
TW5 2TU
Tel: 0784-254041

ASH MEADOW

Dr P F Haimes
Much Hadham Health Centre
Ash Meadow
Herts
SU10 6DE
Tel: 0279-842242

ASHTEAD

Dr F Henari
The Ashtead Hospital
The Warren
Ashtead
Surrey
KT21 2SN
Tel: 0372-276161

ASHTON-UNDER-LYNE

Dr R J Rhodes
Richmond Group Practice
Crickets Lane Health Centre
Ashton-Under-Lyne
Lancs
OL6 6NG
Tel: 061-3399161

ASTON CLINTON

Dr J H Harvey
Acton Clinton Surgery
1 Stablebridge Road
Aston Clinton
HP22 5ND
Tel: 0296-630241

AYLESBURY

RAF Institute of Pathology
and Tropical Medicine
Halton
Aylesbury
Bucks
HP22 5PG
Tel: 0296-623535

Dr M Paul
Bedgrove Health Centre
Jansel Square
Aylesbury
Buckinghamshire
HP21 7ET
Tel: 0296-82737

BALCOMBE

Dr P J Walter
Rapha House Surgery
Stockcroft Road
Balcombe
RH17 6LQ
Tel: 0444-811572

BAMPTON

Dr P J Backhouse
The Surgery
Barnhay
Bampton
Devon
EX16 9NB
Tel: 0398-331304

BANBURY

Dr R Gilchrist
West Bar Surgery
1 West Bar
Banbury
Oxon
OX16 9SF
Tel: 0295-56261

Dr S Heath
The New Surgery
Sibford Gower
Banbury
Oxon
OX15 5RQ
Tel: 0295-78213

BARKING

Dr S N Gupta
7 Salisbury Avenue
Barking
Essex
IG11 9XQ
Tel: 081-5942023

BARNARD CASTLE

Dr F J Hamilton
Barnard Castle Surgery
Victoria Road
Barnard Castle
Co Durham
DL12 8HT
Tel: 690408

BARNET

Dr G N Hanks
Cockfosters Medical Centre
Heddon Court Avenue
Barnet
EN4 9NB
Tel: 081-421137

BARNSLEY

The Health Centre
New Street
Barnsley
South Yorkshire
S70 1LP
Tel: 0226-286122 Ext 3100

Dr M S Littlewood
Surgery
22 Midland Road
Royston
Barnsley
South Yorkshire
S71 4QW
Tel: 0226-727949

Dr M S Littlewood
Surgery
69D Midland Road
Royston
Barnsley
South Yorkshire
S71 4QW
Tel: 0226-722418

Dr N Czepulkowski
The Surgery
48 High Street
Royston
Barnsley
South Yorkshire
S71 4RF
Tel: 0226-722314

BARNSTAPLE

Barnstaple Health Centre
Vicarage Street
Barnstaple
Devon
EX32 7BT
Tel: 0271-71761

Dr C P McCaie
Bear Street Surgery
Health Centre
Vicarage Street
Barnstaple
North Devon
EX32 7BT
Tel: 0271-75221 EXT 214

Dr A Latham
Fremington Medical Centre
11-13 Beards Road
Barnstaple
Devon
EX31 2NT
Tel: 0271-78822

BARROW-IN-FURNESS

Vickers Ltd Medical
    Department
5 Cavendish Park
Barrow-in-Furness
Cumbria
LA14 2SE
Tel: 0229-23366

Dr M C Patel
The Surgery
28-30 Hartington St
Barrow-in-Furness
Cumbria
LA14 5SL
Tel: 0229-870170

Dr A Wiejak
Atkinson Health Centre
Market Street
Barrow-in-Furness
Cumbria
LA14 2LR
Tel: 0229-822205

BARTON

Dr D J Sydenham
The Surgery
Hexton Road
Barton
Bedfordshire
MK45 4TA
Tel: 0582-882050

BARTON HILLS

Bramingham Park Medical
    Centre
Lucas Gardens
Barton Hills
Luton
LU3 4DE
Tel: 0582-597737

BASILDON

Dr P J Kerringan
Laindon Health Centre
Laindon
Basildon
Essex
SS15 5TR
Tel: 0268-46411

Dr R J Bell
West Wing Dipple Medical
    Centre
Wickford Avenue
Pitsea
Basildon
Essex
SS13 3HQ

BASING

Dr J M Fowler
The Hampshire Clinic
Basing Road
Basing
Hampshire

BASINGSTOKE

Out-Patients Department
Basingstoke District Hospital
Park Prewett
Basingstoke
Hants
RG24 9IA

BATH

Bath Clinic
Claverton Dawn Road
Coombe Dawn
Bath
Avon
BA2 7BR

Dr M B Jackson
Oldfield Surgery
45 Upper Oldfield Park
Bath
BA2 3HT
Tel: 0225-421137

Wellcare Health Screening
    Centre
7 Monmouth Place
Off Queen Square
Bath
BA1 2AU

Dr M B Bottomley
The University of Bath
Quarry House
North Road
Clavertondown
Bath
BA2 7AY

Fairfield Park Health Centre
Tyning Lane
Camden Road
Bath
BA1 6EA

Dr R W Gibbs
Grosvenor Surgery
26 Grosvenor Road
London Road
Bath
Avon
BA1 6BA

Dr Conway
Newbridge Surgery
129 Newbridge Hill
Bath
BA1 3PT

BATTLE

Dr T Jardine-Brown
The Surgery
Brede Lane
Sedlescombe
Battle
East Sussex
TN33 OPW

BEACONSFIELD

The Simpson Centre
70 Gregories Road
Beaconsfield
Bucks
HP9 1HL

BECCLES

Dr Ian R Battye
The Health Centre
St Mary's Road
Beccles
Suffolk
NR34 9NQ

BECKENHAM

Ami Sloane Hospital
125 Albermarle Road
Beckenham
Kent
BR3 2HS

Occupational Health Centre
Wellcombe Research
    Laboratory
Langley Court
South Eden Park Road
Beckenham
Kent
BR3 3BS

Dr K P C Carroll
Elm House Surgery
29 Beckenham Road
Beckenham
Kent
BR3 4PR

BEDFORD

Dr J E Hood
Rothesay Surgery
Rothesay House
Rothesay Place
Bedford
MK40 3PX

Dr R Norris
6 Lansdowne Road
Bedford
MK40 2BY

The Surgery
23 De Pary's Avenue
Bedford
MK40 2TX

Dr M Wallis
The Surgery
16 St John's Street
Kempston
Bedford
MK48 8PT

Dr Ian Aldrich
HGS Limited
Occupational Health
    Department
Manton Lane
Bedford
MK41 7PA

Dr B J Crawford
The Surgery
26 Silver Street
Great Barford
Bedford
MK44 3HX

Dr T P Griffith
85 Goldington Avenue
Bedford
MK40 3DB
Tel: 0234 349531

BEDWORTH

Dr C Patel
301 Newtown Road
Bedworth
Warwickshire
CV12 OAJ

BELMONT

Dr D Latham
Sutton Health Clinic
1 Station Approach
Belmont
Sutton
SM2 6DD

BEXHILL-ON-SEA

Dr S P Southwood
Sea Road Surgery
39/41 Sea Road
Bexhill-on-Sea
East Sussex
TN40 1JJ

BEXLEY

Dr M Hoogewerf
Hurst Place Surgery
294A Hurst Road
Bexley
Kent
DA5 3LH

Dr K E Upton
6 Pincotu Road
Bexley Heath
Kent
DA6 7LP
Tel: 081-304 8334

BEXLEY HEATH

Dr K E Upton
6 Pincott Road
Bexley Heath
Kent
DA6 7LP
Tel: 081-304 8334

BICESTER

The Health Centre
Coker Close
Bicester
Oxon
OX6 7AT

BIDEFORE

Dr P J Brummitt
The Wooda Surgery
Clarence Wharf
Barnstaple Street
Bideford
Devon
EX39 4AU

Dr Paul Dean
Bideford Medical Centre
Bideford
North Devon
EX39 3DB

Dr A Latham
The Woodland Clinic
Mines Road
Bideford
Devon
EX32 4BZ

BIGGLESWADE

The Surgery
35-37 The Baulk
Biggleswade
Bedfordshire
SG18 OPX

BILBROOK

Dr A K Woodward
Bilbrook Medical Centre
Brookfield Road
Bilbrook
Wolverhampton
WV8 1DX

BILLERICAY

Dr G Clearhill
The Health Centre
Stock Road
Billericay
Essex
CM12 OBG

BILSTON

Dr A Adma
The Surgery
3 Clifton Street
Hurst Hill
Bilston
West Midlands
WV14 9EY

BIRKENHEAD

Dr M Salahuddin
Old Chester Road Medical
    Centre
241 Old Chester Road
Rock Ferry
Birkenhead
Wirral
L42 3TD

Dr C P Arthur
Claughton Medical Centre
161 Park Road North
Claughton
Birkenhead
L41 0DD

Dr V Dwivedi
Rockferry Health Centre
Bedford Avenue
Birkenhead
Merseyside
L42 4QJ

Dr J W Bates
Oxton Health Centre
40 Balls Road
Birkenhead
Wirral
L43 5RE

BIRMINGHAM

The Medical Room
Birmingham International
    Airport
Birmingham
B26 3QT

The Medical Centre
Craig Croft
Chelmsley Wood
Birmingham
B37 7TR

The Medical Centre
90 Lancaster Street
Birmingham
B4 7AR

British Airways Travel Clinic
100 Church Lane
Handsworth Wood
Birmingham
B20 2ES

Dr S Hasan
Lee Bank Group Practice
10 Bath Row
Lee Bank
Birmingham
West Midlands
B15 1LZ

The Surgery
75-77 Cotterills Lane
Alum Rock
Birmingham
B8 3EZ

Dr F D Hobbs
Bellvue Medical Centre
Edgbaston
Birmingham
B5 7LX
Tel: 021-4402979

Dr V Bathla
143 Albert Road
Hansworth
Birmingham
West Midlands
B21 9LE

Dr D M O'Connell
Priory Dene Private Health
    Centre
Priory Road
Edgbaston
Birmingham
B5 7UG

Dr R C Brake
Poplars Surgery
17 Holly Lane
Erdington
Birmingham
B24 9JN

Dr G J Brown
University Medical Practice
Elms Road
Birmingham
West Midlands
B15 2SE

Dr S S Bakhshi
Travel Vaccination & Medical
    Advisory Centre
127 Soho Hill
Handsworth
Birmingham
B19 1 AT

Dr M Wilkinson
205 Shard End Crescent
Shard End
Birmingham Health Authority
Queen Elizabeth Hospital
Edgbaston
Birmingham
West Midlands
B3 3DH

Yellow Fever Account
Phillip Harris Medical
    Limited
Hazelwell Lane
Stirchley
Birmingham
B30 2PS

Dr M P Allen
The Surgery
57 Woodland Road
Northfield
Birmingham
B31 3HZ

Dr M J McKiernan
Lucas Industries Place
Great King Street
Birmingham
B19 2XF

Dr G S Hayes
The Surgery
43 Old Barn Road
Bournville
Birmingham
B30 1PY

Dr R P Kanas
Medical Department
Cadbury Limited
Bournville
Birmingham
B30 2LU

Dr K Somasundara
21 Salisbury Road
Moseley
Birmingham
B13 8JS

Dr M Forrest
9 Plough and Harrow Road
Edgbaston
Birmingham
B16 8UR

BISHOP AUCKLAND

Dr P Bowron
The Surgery
40 Pinfold Lane
Butterknowle
Bishop Auckland
Co Durham

The Surgery
54 Cockton Hill Road
Bishop Auckland
Co Durham
D14 6BB

The Health Centre
Escomb Road
Bishop Auckland
Co Durham
DL14 6HT

Dr E Eccleston
Braeside Medical Group
The Health Centre
Escomb Road
Bishop Auckland
DL14 6HT

BISHOP'S STORTFORD

Dr J G Schofield
The Surgery
30A Church Street
Bishop's Stortford
Herts
C23 2LY

The Surgery
Station Road
Elsenham
Bishop's Stortford
Herts
CM22 64A

BLACKBURN

Larkhill Health Centre
Mount Pleasant
Blackburn
BB1 5BJ

Little Harwood Health Centre
Plante Tree Road
Blackburn
Lancs
BB1 6PH

BLACKPOOL

The Surgery
155 Newton Drive
Blackpool
Lancs
FY3 8LZ

Dr F T Costello
BUPA Fylde Coast Hospital
St Walburgas Road
Blackpool
Lancs
LY3 8BP

Dr R B Avasthi
Clare Street Medical Centre
194/96 Lytham Road
Blackpool
Lancs
FY1 6EU

BLETCHLEY

Water Eaton Health Centre
Fern Grove
Bletchley
Bucks

BLYTH

Rudley Medical Group
Blyth Health Centre
Blyth
Northumberland

BOGNOR REGIS

Dr A Lean
Felpham & Middleton H/C
109 Flansham Park
Bognor Regis
West Sussex
PO22 6DH

BOLSOVER

Dr M Strelley
The Surgery
Church
Street
Bolsover
Derbyshire
S44 6HB
Tel: 0246-828815

BOLTON

Newlands Medical Centre
Chorley New Road
Bolton
Manchester
BL1 5BP

Kildonan House Group
  Practice
Chorley New Road
Herwick
Bolton
Manchester
BL6 5NW

Dr John Peacock
Stableford Surgery
Church Street
Westhoughton
Bolton
Manchester
BL5 3SF

Dr J A Needham
The Unsworth Group Practice
Captain Lees Road
Westhoughton
Bolton
BL5 3UB

Dr A K Mishra
Pike View Medical Centre
Albert Street
Horwich
Bolton
Gt Manchester

Dr J Thomas
Great Lever Health Centre
Rupert Street
Bolton
Lancs
BL3 6RN

BORDEN

Dr J V Eddey
Pinehill Surgery
Pinehill Road
Borden
Hants
GU35 OBS

Forest Surgery
Chalet Hill
Borden
Hampshire
GU35 ODD

Dr M F Henelly
Woolmer Surgery
Forest Road
Borden
Hampshire
GU35 OBJ

BOREHAMWOOD

Dr J R Longbourne
Fairbrook Medical Centre
Fairway Avenue
Borehamwood
Herts
WD6 1PR
Tel: 081 953 9801

BORROWASH

Dr J G Crompton
207 Victoria Avenue
Borrowash
Derby
DE7 3HG

BOSTON

Dr C Warren
20 Main Ridge West
Boston
Lincolnshire
PE21 6SS

The Surgery
Main Road
Stickley
Boston
Lincs
PE22 8AA

BOURNE END

Dr J M Lloyd Parry
The Hawthornden Surgery
Wharf Lane
Bourne End
Buckinghamshire
SL8 5RX

BOURNEMOUTH

Wintan Health Centre
Alma Road
Winton
Bournemouth
Dorset
BH9 1BP

The Surgery
1628 Wimbourne Road
Kinson
Bournemouth
Dorset
BH11 9AH

Dr J M Beck
Beafort Road Surgery
21 Beafort Road
Southbourne
Bournemouth
Dorset
BH6 5AJ

Dr E S Sylvester
Westbourne Medical Centre
Milburn Road
Bournemouth
Dorset
BH4 9HJ

BOX

Dr J Bullen
Box Surgesy
London Road
Box
Wilts
SN14 9NA

BRACKNELL

Birch Hill Medical Centre
Leppington
Bracknell
Berks
RG12 4WW

BRADFORD

Dr A D Campbell
Leeds Road Hospital
Leeds Road
Bradford
West Yorks
BD3 9LH

Dr A D Campbell
Bradford Royal Infirmary
Occupational Health
Field House
Duckworth Lane
Bradford W Yorks
BD9 6RJ

BRAMHALL

Dr J A Geary
Bramhall Health Centre
Bramhall Lane South
Bramhall
Cheshire
SK7 2DU

BRENTWOOD

The Surgery
The Tile House
33 Shenfield Road
Brentwood
Essex
CM15 8AQ

BRIDLINGTON

The Surgery
35 Wellington Road
Bridlington
E Yorks
YO15 2BA

Dr A J Seeley
Bridlington Medicam
    Practices
North House
7 High Street
Bridgnorth
Shropshire
WV16 4BU

BRIDGWATER

Dr P L D'Ambrumenil
The Surgery
Buckfurleng Farm
Catart
Bridgwater
Somerset
TA7 9HT

Dr Peter Reed
The Surgery
12 Taunton Road
Bridgwater
Somerset
TA6 3LS

BRIGHTON

School Clinic
Morley Street
Brighton
Sussex
BN2 2RH

Dr P A Denis Le Seve
The Health Centre
University of Sussex
Falmer
Brighton
Sussex
BN1 9RW

Dr H Carter & Dr X P N
    Alletamby
4 St Peters Place
Brighton
Sussex
BN1 4SA

BRIGHOUSE

Dr S Farrow
Rydings Hall Surgery
Church Lane
Brighouse
West Yorkshire
HD6 1AT

BRISTOL

The Surgery
Manulife House
10 Marlborough Street
Bristol
Avon
BS1 3NP

Travel Medical Centre Ltd
Charlotte Keel Health Centre
Seymour Road
Bristol
Avon
BS5 OUA

Wellperson Health Services
155 Whiteladies Road
Bristol
Avon
BS8 2RF

The Broadmead Clinic
18 Merchant Street
Bristol
Avon
BS1 3ET

Dr S Bradley
Grange Road Surgery
Bishopsworth
Bristol
BS13 8LD

Dr E J Todd
Bradley Stoke Surgery
Brook Way
Bradley Stoke North
Bristol
BS12 9DS
Tel: 0454 616262

Dr M A Norman
The South Road Surgery
40 South Road
Kingswood
Bristol
BS15 2JQ

Dr J A Bailey
Whiteladies Health Centre
Whatley Road
Clifton
Bristol
Avon
BS8 2PU

Bristol Royal Infirmary
Pharmacy Department
Bristol
Avon
BS9 2PU

Dr T M Southwood/Dr
    Houghton
BrockWay Medical Centre
8 BrockWay
Nailsea
Bristol
Avon
B19 1BZ

Dr J C Watkins
Backwell Medical Centre
15 West Town Road
Backwell
Bristol
Avon
BS19 3HA

Dr S J Fosbury
55 Rayens Cross Road
Long Ashton
Bristol
BS18 9DY

Dr N McCulloch
The Surgery
St Mary Street
Thornbury
Bristol
Avon
BS12 1AA

Nailsea Health Centre
Nailsea
Bristol
Avon
BS19 2EY

Dr K Tremaine
Courtside Surgery
Yate Health Centre
21 West Walk Yate
Bristol
Avon
BS17 4AA

BROADSTAIRS

Reading Road Surgery
235 Beacon Road
Broadstairs
Kent
CT10 3DY

St Peters Surgery
6 Oaklands Avenue
Broadstairs
Kent

BROADSTONE

Dr M I Richardson
Hadleigh House
20 Kirkway
Broadstone
Dorset
BH18 8EE

BROADWAY

Dr T P S Blouch
Barn Close Surgery
40 High Street
Broadway
Worcestershire
WR12 7BT

BROCKENHURST

Dr D S Browne
The Surgery
Highwood Road
Brockenhurst
Hants

BROMLEY

Dr G Ladd
The Surgery
Dysart House
13 Ravensbourne Road
Bromley
Kent
BR1 1HN

BROUGH

The Surgery
60 Welton Road
Brough
North Humberside
HU15 1BH

Dr R A Ferguson
The Health Centre
Gilberdyke
Brough
North Yorkshire
HV15 2U

BUCKHURST HILL

Holly House Hospital
High Road
Buckhurst Hill
Essex
IG9 5HX

The King's Avenue Surgery
23 King's Avenue
Buckhurst Hill
Essex
IG9 5LP

BURFORD

Drs Sharpley, Brown & Wagg
The Surgery
Sheep Street
Burford
Oxon
OX8 4LS

BURNT-ON-THE-WATER

The Surgery
Sherborne Street
Burton-on-the-Water
Gloucestershire
GL54 2BY

BURNT WOOD

Dr L T Harrington
Burntwood Health Centre
Hudson Drive
Burntwood
Staffs
WS7 OEW

BURY

British Airways Travel Clinic
Bury General Hospital
Walmersley Road
Bury
Lancashire
BL9 6PG

Dr M Khan
Peel Health Centre
Angovleme Way
Bury
Lancs
BL9 OBT

BURY ST EDMUNDS

Dr D A Pearson
Woolpit Health Centre
Bury St Edmunds
Suffolk
IP30 9QO

Dr J Cannon
Ixworth Surgery
Peddars Close
Ixworth
Bury St Edmunds
Suffolk
IP31 2HP

Dr R C Robinson
The Guild Hall Surgery
Lower Baxter Street
Bury St Edmunds
Suffolk
IP33 1LE

Dr R C Cooledge
The Surgery
Brittons Road
Barrow
Bury St Edmunds
Suffolk
IP29 5AF

Dr M G Kelvin
Mount Farm Surgery
Lawson Place
Bury St Edmunds
IP32 7EW

Dr C T Dunne
96 Northgate Street
Bury St Edmunds
Suffolk
IP33 1HY

BURNHAM

Dr A R Barrett
Burnham Health Centre
Minniecroft Road
Burnham
Bucks
SL1 7DE

BURNHAM MARKET

Dr F G De L Wright
The Surgery
Church Walk
Burnham Market
King's Lynn
Norfolk
PE31 8DH

BUSHEY HEATH

The Surgery
Rutherford Way
Bushey Heath
Herts
WD2 1NJ

BUXTON

Dr S F King
The Surgery
243 The Square
Buxton
Derbyshire
SK17 6BA

Dr B R Williams
The Stewart Medical Centre
15 Hartington Road
Buxton
Derbyshire
SK17 6JP

Dr A P Briggs
Bath Road Health Centre
Bath Road
Buxton
Derbyshire
SK17 6HL

CAMBERLEY

Dr Hey
The Surgery
143 Park Road
Camberley
Surrey
GU15 2NN

Frimley Green Medical Centre
Beech Road
Frimley Green
Camberley
Surrey
GU16 6QQ

Dr A D Gibb
37 Upper Gordon Road
Camberley
Surrey
GU15 2HJ

Dr S J Jones
Hartley Corner
51 Frogmore Road
Blackwater
Camberley
Surrey
GU17 0DB

CAMBOURNE

Dr S R Barton
Veor Surgery
South Terrace
Cambourne
Cornwall
TR14 8SN

CAMBRIDGE

Addenbrooke's Hospital
Hills Road
Cambridge
Essex
CB2 2QQ

BA Travel Clinic
1 Huntingdon Road
Cambridge
Essex

Dr P Niemczuk
281 Mill Road
Cambridge
CB1 3DG

Dr J Owens
56 Trumpington Street
Cambridge
CB2 1RG

Arbury Road Surgery
114 Arbury Road
Cambridge
Essex
CB4 2JG

Dr R B Church
Shelford Health Centre
Ashen Green
Great Shelford
Cambridge
CB2 5EY
Tel: 0223-843661

Dr P D Toase
1 Huntingdon Road
Cambridge
CB3 0DB
Tel: 0223-64127

CANNOCK

Surgery
65 Church Street
Cannock
Staffs
WS11 1DS

CANTERBURY

Dr A Otati
Early Care Health
Screening Centre
Canterbury
Kent
CT1 3TB

The Chaucer Hospital
Nackington Road
Canterbury
Kent
CT4 7AR

Dr H Byrom
Cossington House Surgery
Cossington Road
Canterbury
Kent
CT1 3HX

Dr D M Jones
Bridge Surgery
Green Court
Bridge
Canterbury
Kent
CT4 5LU

CARLISLE

The Central Clinic
Victoria Place
Carlisle
CA1 1HN

CARNFORTH

Dr Simon Kaye
Green Close Surgery
Kirkby Lonsdale
Carnforth
Lancs
LA6 2BS

CARTERTON

The Surgery
17 Alvescot Road
Carterton
Oxfordshire
OX8 2JL

CASTLE DONNINGTON

The Surgery
53 Borough Road
Castle Donnington
Derby
DE7 2LB

CASTLEFORD

Dr G R Aldridge
Riverside Medical Centre
Savile Road
Castleford
West Yorkshire
WF10 1PH

CATERHAM

Dr C S Wood
The Surgery
Caterham Hill Clinic
Chaldon Road
Caterham
Surrey
CR3 5PH

Dr F C O'Brien
Town End Surgery
41 Town End
Caterham
CR3 5UJ

CHALFONT ST GILES

Dr J L Cosgrove
St Giles Surgery
Townfield Lane
Chalfont St Giles
Bucks
HP8 4QF

CHARTHAM

Dr D Kinnersley
The Surgery
Parish Road
Chartham
Canterbury
Kent
CT4 7JU

Principal Pharmacist
Garlands Hospital
Carlisle
Cumbria
CA1 2SX

The Treasurer
East Cumbria Health
    Authority
13-14 Portland
Square
Carlisle
Cumbria
CA1 1PT

CHEADLE

AMI Alexandra Hospital
Mill Lane
Cheadle
Cheshire
SK8 2PX

Dr J R Adams
Cheadle Medical Practice
1-5 Ashfield Crescent
Cheadle
Cheshire
SK8 1BH

NORTH CHEAM

St Anthony's Hospital
London Road
North Cheam
Surrey
SM3 5DW

CHEDDAR

Dr Blakeney-Edward
Cheddar Medical Centre
Roynan Way
Cheddar
Somerset
BA27 3NZ

CHELFORD

Chelford Surgery
Elmstead Road
Chelford
Nr Macclesfield
Cheshire
SK11 9BS

CHELMSFORD

The Medical Centre
Ground Floor Block A
County Hall
Chelmsford
Essex
CM1 1LX

CHELTENHAM

Windrush Medical Centre
Laverham House
77 St George's Place
Cheltenham
Gloucestershire
GL50 3PP

Dr M Lewis
Dowty Group
Medical Services
Arle Court
Cheltenham
Glos
GL51 OTP

The Surgery
Bakery Crescent
St George's Place
Cheltenham
Gloucestershire
GL54 2BY

CHERTSEY

Dr J B Sales
Family Health Centre
Stepgates
Chertsey
Surrey

Dr P F Brodribb
Family Health Centre
Stepgates
Chertsey
Surrey
KT16 8HY

CHESHAM

The New Surgery
Lindo Close
Chesham
Bucks
HP5 2JP

CHESTER

Garden Lane Medical Centre
19 Garden Lane
Chester
Cheshire
CH1 4EN

Northgate Medical Centre
10 Upper Northgate Street
Chester
Cheshire
CH1 4EE

Upton Village Surgery
Wealstone Lane
Chester
Cheshire
CH2 1HD

Dr C R Lewis
Park Medical Centre
Shavington Avenue
Newton Lane
Heale Chester
Cheshire
CH2 3RD

Dr M Griffiths
Boughton Health Centre
Hoole Lane
Chester
Cheshire
LH2 3DP

Dr H D Charles-Jones
Upton Lodge Surgery
Wealstone Lane
Upton
Chester
Cheshire
CH2 1HD

Dr P Bradley
Lache Health Centre
Hawthorn Road
Chester
CH 8HX
Tel: 0244-671991

CHESTER-LE-STREET

Dr W A Duke
Bridge End Surgery
Chester-le-Street
Co Durham
DH3 3SL

CHESTERFIELD

The Health Centre
Saltergate
Chesterfield
Derbyshire
S40 1SY

Chatsworth Road Medical
   Centre
Chatsworth Road
Brampton
Chesterfield
S40 3JX

Dr P R Aldred
Hich Street Medical Centre
19 High Street
Staveley
Chesterfield
Derbyshire
S43 3UU

Dr A K Sharma
The Medical Centre
1 Tennyson Avenue
Saltergate
Chesterfield
S40 4SN

Dr I R Serrell
Ash Lodge
73 Old Road
Brampton
Chesterfield
Derbyshire

CHESSINGTON

Dr A J Lyons
207 Hook Road
Chessington
Surrey
KT9 1EA

CHICHESTER

The Medical Centre
Cawley Road
Chichester
West Sussex
PO19 1 XT

CHIPPENHAM

Jubliee Field Surgery
Yatton Keynell
Chippenham
Wiltshire
SN13 7EJ

Dr A T Wright
The Surgery
47 Marshfield Road
Chippenham
Wiltshire
SN15 1JU

CHIPPING NORTON

West Street Surgery
12 West Street
Chipping Norton
Oxfordshire
OX7 5AA

CHISLEHURST

Dr R W May
The Surgery
42 High Street
Chislehurst
Kent
BR7 5AX

CHOPPINGTON

Guide Post Medical Group
North Parade
Choppington
Northumberland
NE62 5RA

CHORLEY

Dr S N Hilton
Cunliff Medical Centre
41 Cunliffe
Chorley
Lancashire
PR7 2BA

Dr D M McAllister
The Surgery
Granville Street
Adlington
Chorley
PR6 9PY
Tel: 0757-481917

CHORLEY WOOD

The Elms Surgery
7 Lower Road
Chorley Wood
Hertsordshire
WD3 5EA

CINDERFORD

Dr D Shan
Forest Health Centre
Dockham Road
Cinderford
Gloucestershire
GL14 2AN

CIRENCESTER

The Park Surgery
Old Tetbury Road
Cirencester
Gloucestershire
GL7 1US

Dr C M Marriott
The Surgery
1 The Avenue
Cirencester
Gloucestershire
GL7 1EH

CLACTON-ON-SEA

Dr G A Sweeney
The Surgery
Ranworth
103 Pier Avenue
Clacton-on-sea
Essex
CO15 1NJ

CLAYGATE

Dr R Leary
17 Torrington Road
Claygate
Surrey
KT10 0SA

CLECKHEATEN

Dr G S Fox
The Health Centre
Greenside
Cleckheaten
West Yorks
BD19 5AP

CLITHEROE

Dr R J Higson
Clitheroe Health Centre
Railway View Avenue
Clitheroe
Lancs
BB7 2JH

CLIFTON HAMPDEN

Drs E A Meinhard & R H
    Lynch-Bloss
The Surgery
Watery Lane
Clifton Hampden
Oxon
OX14 3EL

CODSALL

Dr A Plant
The Surgery
Bakers Way
Codsall
Wolverhampton
WV8 1HD

COLCHESTER

The Surgery
Priory House
St Botolph's Street
Colchester
Essex
CO2 7EA

The Surgery
Birch
Colchester
Essex
CO2 0NL

Dr A D Snell
7 Rectory Road
Rowhedge
Colchester
CO5 7HP

Dr F Ayache
The Surgery
56 Richardsons Road
East Bergholt
Colchester
CO7 6RP
Tel: 0206 298272

COBHAM

Dr G Winter
The Health Centre
Downsidebridge Road
Cobham
KT11 1AE

Dr L Rushbrook
Layer Road Surgery
Layer Road
Colchester
Essex
CO2 9LA

CONGLETON

Readesmoor GP Practice
29/29A West Street
Congleton
Cheshire
CW12 1JN

CORBY

Dr D A Palmer
The Medical Centre
9 Elizabeth Street
NN17 1SJ
Tel: 0536-202508

CORRINGHAM

Dr A Rigg-Miller
Lake House
72 Fobbing Road
Corringham
SS17 9JD

CORSHAM

Dr R C F Drummond
The Porch
33 High Street
Corsham
Wiltshire
SN13 0EY

COSHAM

Cosham Health Centre
Velvis Way
Cosham
Portsmouth
Hampshire
PO6 3AW

COVENTRY

Hillfield Health Centre
1 Howard Street
Coventry
West Midlands
CV1 4GH

Dr G S Judge
Corsewood Medical Centre
95 Momus Boulevard
Coventry
CV2 5NB
Tel: 0203-457497

Communicable Disease
    Control
Edyvean Walker Ward
Gulson Hospital
Gulson Road
Coventry

Dr I MacDonald
Allesley Village Surgery
163 Birmingham Road
Allesley
Coventry
West Midlands
CV8 1ET

Dr H C Evans
The Surgery
2 Maidevale Crescent
Coventry
West Midlands
CV3 6FZ

Dr N Greenhalgh
Holbrook Health Centre
Holbrook Lane
Coventry
West Midlands
CV6 4DG

Dr P T Dooley
1A Engleton Road
Radford
Coventry
CV6 1JF

Dr R J Ballantine
University of Warwick
Health Centre
Coventry
West Midlands
CV4 7AL

Dr A A Ezzat
Park Road Medical
35 Park Road
Coventry
West Midlands
CV1 2LA

Dr G Cooper
Woodside Medical Centre
Jardine Crescent
Coventry
West Midlands
CV4 9PL

Dr P J Horn
The Surgery
2 Bennetts Road
North Keresley End
Nr Coventry
West Midlands
CV7 8LA

CRAMLINGTON

Dr A P Dove
Brockwell Medical Group
Brockwell Centre
Northumbrian Road
Cramlington
Northumberland
NE23 9XZ

CRANBROOK

Dr H Butler
The Surgery
Orchard End
Dorothy Avenue
Cranbrook
Kent
TN17 3AY

CRANLEIGH

Dr H Butler
The Surgery
Orchard End
Dorothy Avenue
Cranbrook
Kent
TN17 3AY

The Health Centre
Cranleigh
Surrey
GU6 8AE

CRAWLEY

Dr A L Cooper
Bridge Medical Centre
Wassand Close
Three Bridges Road
Crawley
Sussex
RH10 1LL
Tel: 0293-536025

CREWE

Moss Lane Surgery
Moss Lane
Nr Crewe
Cheshire
CW3 9NQ

NR CREWE

Moss Lane Surgery
Moss Lane
Madeley
Near Crewe
Cheshire
CW3 9NQ

Dr B S Tate
Hunderford Road Surgery
Crewe
Cheshire
CW1 1EQ

CROWBOROUGH

Dr P C Cobb
The Surgery
Saxonbury House
Croft Road
Crowborough
East Sussex
TN6 1DP

CROYDON

Dr K P Walker
Eexecutive Medical Centre
24 Chatsworth Road
Croydon
Surrey
CR0 1HA

The Surgery Suite 3
15 Crown Hill
Church Street
Croydon
London
CR0 1RY

Dr A Nawrocki
The Surgery
5961 Addiscombe Road
Croydon
Surrey
CR0 6SD

CRUMPSALL

Dr P A Dixon
The Surgery
53-55 Crescent Road
Crumpsall
Manchester
M8 7JT

CUFFLEY

Dr C P J Taylor
The Health Centre
Maynard Place
Cuffley
Hertfordshire
EN6 4JA

DAGENHAM

Occupational Health
    Department
Rhone-Roter Ltd
Rainham Road South
Dagenham
Essex
RM10 7XS

DARTFORD

Dr D Jones
Dartford West Health Centre
Tower Road
Dartford
Kent
DA1 2HA

DANENTRY

Abbey House Surgery
Golding Close
Daventry
Northamptonshire
NN11 5RA

DEAL

Dr N J Sharvill
1 Victoria Road
Deal
Kent
CT14 7AU

DERBY

Dr K C Patel
Littleover Surgery
640 Burton Surgery
Littleover
Derby
DE3 6EL

Dr P J Horden
The Surgery
233 Village Street
Derby
DE3 8DD

The Clinic
Cathedral Road
Derby
Derbyshire
DE1 3PE

Dr D Cooke
Riversdale Surgery
59 Bridge Street
Belper
Derby
DE5 1AY
Tel: 0773-822386

Derbyshire Area Health
    AUTH
South Derbyshire District
118 Osmaston Road
Derby
Derbyshire

The Medical Centre
Two Dales
Nr Matlock
Derbyshire

Dr J P B Budgen
Osmaston Surgery
212 Osmaston Road
Derby
Derbyshire
DE3 8JX

Dr G A Richmond
The Surgery
Limes Avenue
Alfreton
Derby
Derbyshire
DE5 7DW

Dr J M Rossiter
Alvaston Medical Centre
14 Boulton Lane
Alvaston
Derbyshire
DE2 0GE

Dr J Spincer
The Surgery
53 Harrington Street
Normanton
Derbyshire
DE3 8PH

Dr J Spincer
The Surgery Oakwood Med/
    Centre
Danebridge Crescent
Oakwood
Derby
Derbyshire
DE2 2HT

Dr R Edyvean
Derwent Medical Centre
26 North Street
Derby
DE1 3AZ

Dr J Blissett
Park Lane Surgery
2 Park Lane
Allestree
Derby
DE3 2DS
Tel: 0332 552461

Dr A Hough
Wilson Street Surgery
11 Wilson Street
Derby
DE1 1PG
Tel: 0332 326628

DEVIZES

Dr Elizabeth Madigan
The Lansdowne Surgery
Waiblingen Way
Devizes
Wiltshire
SN10 2BU

DIDCOT

Mereland Road Surgery
17-19 Mereland Road
Didcot
Oxon
OX11 8AS

DIDSBURY

Medical Surgery
599 Wilmslow Road
Didsbury
Manchester
M20 9QT

DONCASTER

The Health Clinic
Chequer Road
Doncaster
DN1 2PW

Dr R J Wyatt
Misterton Group Practice
March Lane
Misterton
Doncaster
DN10 4DP

DORCHESTER

The Surgery
South Lodge
South Walks
Dorchester
Dorset
DT1 1DS

DOVERCOURT

Dovercourt Health Clinic
Dovercourt
Harwich
Essex
CO12 4ET

DOWNHAM MARKET
    DIFFIELD

The Surgery
The Towers
Downham Market
Norfolk
PE38 9AF

Dr I A Jollie
The Surgery
Beeford
Driffield
YO25 8BA

DROITWICH-SPA

The Health Centre
Droitwich-Spa
Worcestershire
WR9 8RD

DUNSTABLE

The Health Centre
Priory Gardens
Church Street
Dunstable
Beds
LU6 1SF

Dr C Quartly
West Street Surgery
89 West Street
Dunstable
Bedfordshire
LU6 1SF

DUNMOW

Dr J S B Jackson
Road End Surgery
6A Stortford Road
Dunmow
Essex
CM6 1DB

DURHAM

Cheveley Park Medical Centre
Belmont
Durham
DH1 2UW

Dr J W Charters
University of Durham
42 Old elvet
Durham
DH1 3JF

Appendix 1

EALING

Ealing Hospital Traval Clinic
Pasteur Suite
Ealing Hospital
Uxbridge Road
Middlesex
UB1 3HW

EASTBOURNE

The Arlington Road Medical
   Practice
1 Arlington Road
Eastbourne
East Sussex
BN21 1DH

EAST BRIDGFORD

Dr R O B Scaffardi
Medical Centre
87 Main Street
East Bridgford
Nottingham
NG13 8NH

EAST GRINSTEAD

The Practice
Judges Close
East Grinstead
Sussex
TH19 3AR

Moatfield Surgery
St Michael's Road
East Grinstead
W Sussex
R19 2GW

EASTHAM

Dr S Williams
The Eastham Group Practice
170 Plymyard Avenue
Eastham
Wirral
L62 8EH

EAST HORSLEY

Dr P Morazzi
Medical Centre
Kingston Avenue
East Horsley
Surrey
KT24 6QT

EASTLEIGH

Dr J Gibson
Stokewood Surgery
Fairoak Road
Fairoak
Eastleigh
SO5 7LU

EAST MOSELEY

Dr M Parry
Central Surgery
15 Seymour Road
East Molesey
Surrey
KT8 0PB

EAST PRESTON

The Surgery
35 Worthing Road
East Preston
East Sussex
BN16 1BG

EAST TILBURY

Dr A Rigg-Milner
The Medical Centre
Princess Margaret's Road
East Tilbury
RM18 8RL

Dr R S Kahn
East Tilbury Health Centre
85 Coronation Avenue
East Tilbury
Essex
RM18 8SW
Tel: 0375-846232

The Surgery
3 Bure
East Tilbury
Essex
RM18 8SF

EASTWOOD

Dr T D Lester
The Surgery
Church Walk
Eastwood
Nottingham
NG16 3BH

ECCLESFIELD

Dr R Oliver
Ecclesfield Group Practice
Mill Road
Ecclesfield
Sheffield
S30 3XQ

EDGEHILL

Dr Shiv Pande
14 North View
Edgehill
Liverpool
L7 8TS

EDGWARE

Dr C D Korn
The Surgery
104A Stag Lane
Edgware
Middlesex
HA8 5LW

Dr A Cohen
The Bacon Lane Surgery
11 Bacon Lane
Edgware
Middlesex
HA8 5AT

Dr M T Wyndham
Lane End House
25 Edgwarebury Lane
Edgware
Middlesex

Dr M Ferris
Lane End House
25 Edgwarebury Lane
Edgware
Middlesex
HA8 8LJ

EGREMONT

Dr J Veitch
Beech House Group Practice
Main Street
Edgremont
Cumbria
CA22 2DB

ELSTREE

Sshopwick Surgery
Everett Court
Romeland
Elstree
Hertfordshire
WD6 3BJ

ELLESMERE PORT

Dr J Stringer
Group Practice Surgery
Chester Road
Whitby
Ellesmere Port
South Wirral
L65 6TG

EMSWORTH

Dr D L ingram
Emsworth Surgery
6 North Street
Emsworth
PO10 7DD

ENFIELD

Dr M Gocman
The Surgery
70 Silver Street
Enfield
Middlesex
EN1 3EB

Eagle House Surgery
291 High Street
Enfield
Middlesex
EN3 4DN

Charlton House Surgery
28 Tenniswood Road
Enfield
Middlesex
EN1 3LL

ENGLEFIELD GREEN

The Health Centre
Bond Street
Englefield Green
Surrey
TW20 0PF

EPSOM

Dr J S Senhenn
Bourne Hall Health Centre
Ewell
Epsom
Surrey
KT17 1TG
Tel: 081-3942367

ESHER

Littleton Surgery
33 Esher Park Avenue
Esher
Surrey
KT10 9NY

EXETER

Principal Pharmacist
Royal D & E Hospital
Barrack Road
Exeter
EX2 5DW

Dr K Thomas
Student Health Centre
Reed Mews
Streatham Drive
Exeter
EX4 4QP

Dr C S Reaves
Charter Surgery
38 Polsloe Road
Exeter
EX1 2DW

Dr V C E Rosser
Heavitree Health Court
South Lawn Terrace
Heavitree
Exeter
EX1 2RX

Dr D H McFadyen
Mount Pleasant Health Centre
Exeter
Devon
EX4 6EL
Tel: 0392-55722

Dr K J Bolden
Mount Pleasant Health Centre
Mount Pleasant Road
Exeter
EX4 7BW
Tel: 0392 55262

FAIRFORD

Dr M J G Knights
Hillary Cottage Surgery
Keblelawns
Fairford
Gloucestershire
GL7 4BQ

FALLOWFIELD

Dr S L Goodman
Ladybarn Group Practice
177 Mauldeth Road
Fallowfield
Manchester
M14 6SG

FALMOUTH

Dr R V Webster
The Health Centre
Trevaylor Road
Falmouth
Gloucestershire
TR11 2LH

FAKENHAM

Fareham Surgery
Greenway Lane
Fakenham
Norfolk
NR21 8ET

FAREHAM

Dr L J Palmer
The Health Centre
Osborn Road
Fareham
Hampshire
PO16 7ER

Dr A P Wolpe
The Surgery
187 Gudgeheath Lane
Fareham
Hampshire
PO15 6QA

FARNBOROUGH

Summerlands Surgery
Starts Hill Road
Farnborough
Kent
BR6 7AR

Dr Vinod Kumar
North Camp Surgery
31 Alexandra Road
Farnborough
Hampshire
GU14 6BS

FAVERSHAM

Dr A J Taylor
The Health Centre
Bank Street
Faversham
Kent
ME13 8PR

Dr R Kesson
Faversham Health Centre
Bank Street
Faversham
Kent
ME13 8PR

FELIXSTOWE

Dr B M G Clarke
Central Surgery
201 Hamilton Road
Felixstowe
Suffolk
IP11 7DT

FLEET

Dr N A D Clark
The Surgery
Branksomewood Road
Fleet
Hampshire
GU13 8JX

FOLKESTONE

Dr M A A M Fernandes
The Manor Clinic
31 Manor Road
Folkstone
Kent
CT20 2SE

Dr J Chappell
White House Surgery
1 Cheriton High Street
Folkestone
Kent
CT19 4PU

Dr Y Y Amin
Central Surgery
86 Cheriton Road
Folkestone
Kent
CT20 2QH

Dr D P Evans
The New Surgery
128 Canterbury Road
Folkestone
Kent
CT19 5NR

FORMBY

Dr S J Crosby
Village Surgery
Elbow Lane
Formby
Liverpool
L37 4AW

GAINSBOROUGH

Dr M Nicklin
3 Caskgate Street Surgery
Gainsborough
Lincs
DN21 2QL

Dr C M Woragg
The New Surgery Traingate
Kirton
Lindsey
Nr Gainsborough
Lincolnshire
DN21 4DG

GALGATE

Dr R G Jackson
Health Centre
Highland Brow
Galgate
LA2 ONB

GATESHEAD

Glenpark Medical Centre
Ravensworth Road
Durston
Gateshead
NE11 9AD

Dr G J Penrice
Denewell House
Denewell Avenue
Gateshead
Tyne and Wear
NE9 5HD

GATWICK

BA Travel Clinic
London (Gatwick) Airport
Grawley
Sussex
RH10 2FH

Dr P J Chapman
Airport Medical Services
Penta Hotel Medical Suite
Gatwick Airport
Horley
Surrey
RH6 OBE

Gatwick Medical Services
South Terminal Medical
  Centre
London (Gatwick) Airport
West Sussex
RH6 ONP

Dr D Tallent
Dan Air Services Ltd
Newman House
Victoria Road
Horley
Surrey
RH6 7QC

Safety Regulation Group
Civil Aviation Authority
Aviation House
South Area
Gatwick Airport
West Sussex
RH6 OYR

Dr J P G Spencer
GAL Occupational Health
  Service
Ashdown House
Gatwick Airport
West Sussex
RH6 ONP

GLASTONBURY

The Glastonbury Surgery
Feversham Lane
Glastonbury
Somerset
BA6 9LP

GILLINGHAM

Occupational Health Service
Medway Hospital
Windmill Road
Gillingham
Kent

GLEDHOLT

Dr J A Birstow
The Surgery
Clevelands
3 Westbourne Road
Gledholt
Huddersfield
HD1 4LB

GLOSSOP

Peak Health Vaccination
  Centre
Manor Street
Glossop
Derbyshire
SK13 7PS

GLOUCESTER

Gloucestershire Royal
  Hospital
Great Western Road
Gloucester
Gloucestershire
GL1 3NN

Dr M Lewis
Dowty Rotol Ltd
Cheltenham Road
Gloucester
Gloucestershire
GL2 9QH

Dr R P Norwich
The Clinic
19 College Green
Gloucester
Gloucestershire
GL1 2ER

Dr J Steele
The Surgery
42 The Street
Uley
Dursley
Gloucester
Gloucestershire
GL11 6AW

Dr M F Lewis
The Surgery
77 Church Street
Tewkesbury
Gloucester
Gloucestershire
GL20 5RY

GODALMING

Dr R M Butcher
The Square Medical Practice
High Street
Godalming
GU7 1AZ

GOSPORT

Dr D A Evans
Gosport Health Centre
Gosport
Hampshire
PO12 3PN

Dr P P Garratt
151 Stoke Road
Gosport
Hampshire
PO12 1SF
Tel: 0705 581529

GODSTONE

Dr C W Howard
Ponnt Tail
The Green
Godstone
Surrey
RH9 8DY
Tel: 0883 742279

GRANTHAM

The Surgery
Colsterworth
Grantham
Lincolnshire
BG33 5NJ

GRAVESEND

The Surgery
30 Old Road West
GravesEnd
Kent
DA11 OLL

GRAYS

Dr A J Rigg-Milner
111 Orsett Road
Grays
Essex
RM17 5HA

GREAT MISSENDEN

AMI Chiltern Hospital
Great Missenden
Buckinghamshire
HP16 OEN

The Surgery
3 Chequers Drive
Prestwood
Great Missenden
Buckinghamshire
HP16 9DU

Dr P R Barker
Prospect House Surgery
High Street
Great Missenden
Buckinghamshire
HP16 0BG

GREAT SUTTON

Group Practice Centre
Old Chester Road
Great Sutton
South Wirral
L66 3PB

GREAT YARMOUTH

North Sea Medical Centre Ltd
3 Lowestoft Road
Gorleston-on-Sea
Great Yarmouth
Norfolk
NR31 6SG

Dr H MacDonald Taylor
Hemsby Medical Centre
1 King's Court
Hemsby
Great Yarmouth
Norfolk
NR29 4EW

GREEN HAMMERTON

Dr R N R Simpson
Springbank Surgery
York Road
Green Hammerton
York
North Yorkshire
YO5 8BN

GREENFORD

Occupational Health
Glaxo Group Research
    Limited
Greenford Road
Greenford
Middlesex
UB6 0HE

Dr N H Segall
Oldfield Family Practice
285 Greenford Road
Greenford
Middlesex
UB6 8RA

GRIMSBY

The Clinic
34 Dudley Street
Grimsby
South Humberside
DN31 1QQ

The Surgery
Worsley Road
Immingham
Grimsby
South Humberside
DN40 1BE

Grimsby District General
    Hospital
Scartho Road
Grimsby
South Humberside
DU33 2BA

Dr K S Trivedi
The Surgery
500 Cromwell Road
Grimsby
South Humberside
DN37 9JY

Dr J Warren
The Surgery
2 Littlefield Lane
Grimsby
South Humberside
DN31 2LG

GUILDFORD

Robens Institute
Occupational Health Service
30 Occam Road
University of Surrey
Guildford
Surrey
HU2 5YW

The Guildford Medical Centre
1 Commercial Road
Guildford
Surrey
GU2 4SU

New Inn Surgery
202 London Road
Guildford
Surrey
GY4 7JS

Dr G R Tyrell
Shere Surgery and Dispensary
Shere
Guildford
Surrey
GU5 9HN

Dr J Beaumont
ST Nicholas Surgery
Bury Street
Guildford
Surrey
GU2 5AW

Dr D R Elliott
The Surgery
56 Epsom Road
Guildford
Surrey
GU3 3LE

The Surgery
The Street
Wonersh
Guildford
Surrey
GU5 0PE

Woodbridge Hill Surgery
1 Deerbarn Road
Guildford
Surrey
GU2 6AT

HADDENHAM

Haddenham Health Centre
Banks Road
Haddenham
Bucks
HP17 8EE

HADLEIGH

Dr D Smithson
The Hollies GP Surgery
41 Rectory Road
Hadleigh
Essex
SS7 2NA

Dr J N Flather
Health Centre
Market Place
Hadleigh
Suffolk
IP7 5DN

HALESFIELD

Telford and District
Occupational Health Service
Health Centre
Halesfield 13
Telford
Salop
TF7 4QP

HALESOWEN

Dr R A Johnson
Halesowen Health Centre
14 Birmingham Street
Halesowen
West Midlands
B63 3HL

HALIFAX

Dr C M Wigley
Stannary House Surgery
Stainland
Halifax
West Yorkshire
HX4 9HA

Dr R T Brown
KOS Clinic
Roylands Street
Hipperholme
Halifax
West Yorkshire
HX3 8AF

HAMILTON

Dr C P Stewart
Dr P C M Barton
74 Portland Place
Hamilton
Midlands

HARLOW

Harlow Industrial Health
    Service
Edinburgh House
Edinburgh Way
Harlow
Essex
CM20 2DG

Dr J Radix
Barbara Castle Health Centre
Broadley Road
Harlow
Essex
CM19 5SJ

Dr K N Tully
Keats House
Bush Fair
Harlow
Essex
CM18 6LY
Tel: 0279 444404

HARPENDEN

Dr D P Tominey
The Surgery
3 Thompson's Close
Harpenden
Hertford
Hertfordshire
AL5 4ES

HARROGATE

Dr M A Scatchard
51A Leeds Road
Harrogate
HG2 8AY
Tel: 0423-566636

HARROW

British Airways Travel Clinic
Harrow Health Care Centre
84-88 Pinner Road
Harrow
Middlesex
HA1 4LF

Lanfranc Court Surgery
2 Lanfranc Court
Greenford Road
Harrow
Middlesex
HA1 3QE

Dr J M Justice
Simpson Home Medical
    Centre
255 Eastcote Lane
Harrow
Middlesex
HA2 8RS

The Surgery
196 Pinner Road
Harrow
Middlesex
HA1 4NS

Dr Dilip C Patel
The Surgery
18 Bethecar Road
Harrow
Middlesex
HA1 1SE

Dr G A Golden
The Surgery
369 Kenton Road
Harrow
Middlesex
HA3 0XF

Appendix 1

HARTLEPOOL

Dr A R Dawson
456 West View Road
Hartlepool
Cleveland
TS24 9LW

HARWICH

Dover Court Health Centre
407 Main Road
Dover Court
Harwich
Essex
CO12 4ET

HASLEMERE

Dr A Thomas
Haslemere Health Centre
Church Lane
Haslemere
Surrey
GU27 2BQ

HASLINGDEN

Dr M M A Badr
The Surgery
7-9 Manchester Road
Haslingden
Lancashire
BB4 5SL

HASTINGS

Dr M J Metson
The Surgery
164 Harold Road
Hastings
East Sussex
TN35 5NH

HATCH END

Dr C S Jenner
The Surgery
118 Uxbridge Road
Hatch End
Middlesex
HA5 4DS

HATFIELD

The Surgery
Lister House
The Common
Hatfield
Hertfordshire
AL20 0NL

Medical Department
British Aerospace Aircraft
    Group
Comet Way
Hatfield
Hertfordshire
AL10 9TL

HAVERHILL

Dr C A Cornish
Christmas Maltings Surgery
Camps Road
Haverhill
Suffolk

HAWKHURST

Dr J Clewis
The Surgery
North Ridge
Rye Road
Hawkhurst
Kent
TN18 4EX

HAXBY

Dr A L Harris
Haxby Health Centre
Haxby
York
YO3 3PL

HAYDON BRIDGE

Dr S D Ford
Haydon Bridge Health Centre
North Bank
Haydon Bridge
Northumberland
NE47 6HG

HAYWARDS HEATH

Dr P J Dawson
Dolphins Practice
The Health Centre
Heath Road
Haywards Heath
West Sussex
RH16 3BB

HEATHFIELD

Dr S M Wadman
The Surgery
96-98 High Street
Heathfield
East Sussex
TN21 8JD

HEBDEN BRIDGE

Dr S R Kay
Hebden Bridge Health Centre
Hangingroyd Lane
Hebden Bridge
HX7 6AG

HEMEL HEMPSTEAD

Dr Toorawa
Lincoln House Surgery
Wolsey Road
Hemel Hempstead
Hertfordshire
HP2 4SH

Dr R M J Price
The Surgery
Parkwood Drive
Hemel Hempstead
Hertfordshire
HP1 2LD

BP Oil UK Limited
BP House Breakspear Road
Hemel Hempstead
Hertfordshire
HP2 4UL

Dr F M Hirji
Grove Hill Medical Centre
Kilbridge Court
Grove Hill
Hemel Hempstead
Hertfordshire
HP2 6AP

HENLEY-ON-THAMES

Dr Melhuish
The New Surgery
York Road
Henley-on-Thames
Oxon
RG9 2DR

The Surgery
Nettlebed
Henley-on-Thames
Oxon
RG9 5AK

Dr C R Purvis
The Hart Practice
York Road
Henley-on-Thames
RG9 2DR
Tel: 0491 572264

HEREFORD

Dr P J Matthews
The Surgery
Moorfield House
Hereford

Dr A E Cutler
County Hospital,
    Occupational Health
    Department
Hereford
HR1 2GR

HERNE BAY

Dr P Samsworth
St Anne's Surgery
161 Station Road
Herne Bay
Kent
CT6 5NF

HESSLE

Dr Rennie T Joseph
The Practice
2A Booth Ferry Road
Hessle
North Humberside
HU13 9AY

HESTON

Dr M R Turner
Skyways Medical Centre
2 Shelley Crescent
Heston
Middlesex
TW5 9BJ

HIGHWORTH

Dr C R Lloyd
Westrop Surgery
Highworth
Wiltshire
SN6 7DN

HIGHFIELD

Dr D J Newton
Highfield Surgery
Highfield Way
Hazlemere
High Wycombe
HP15 7UN

HIGH WYCOMBE

The Surgery
Valley Road
Hughenden
High Wycombe
Buckinghamshire
HP14 4LG

Dr P T Fox
Wye Valley Surgery
2 Desborough Avenue
High Wycombe
Buckinghamshire
HP11 2RN

Dr G Livingston
Wycombe General Hospital
Occupational Health
Queen Alexandra Road
High Wycombe
Buckinghamshire
HP11 2TT

Dr R Reiey
The Surgery
65 Desborough Avenue
High Wycombe
Buckinghamshire
HP11 2SD

HILDENBOROUGH

The Hildenborough Medical
    Group
79 Tonbridge Road
Hildenborough
Kent
TN11 9BH

HINDHEAD

Dr F J Lecouilliard
Grayshott Surgery
Boundary Road
Hindhead
Surrey
GU26 6TY

HITCHIN

The Surgery
Regal Chambers
50 Bancroft
Hitchin
Hertfordshire
SG5 1JZ

HODDESDON

The Limes Surgery
8-14 Limes Court
Conduit Lane
Hoddesdon
Hertfordshire
EN11 8BE

Dr A Muigherjee
The Surgery
Groom Road
Purnford
Hoddesdon
Hertfordshire
EN10 6BW

The Amwell Street Surgery
19 Amwell Street
Hoddesdon
Hertfordshire
EN11 8TU

HOLMFRITH

Dr J R Clayden
Elmwood Health Centre
Huddersfield Road
Holmfrith
HD7 2TT

HORLEY

Airport Medical Services
Gatwick Penta Hotel
Povcy Cross Road
Horley Surgery
RH6 0BE

HORNCHURCH

The Surgery
Marylands
Hornchurch Road
Hornchurch
Essex
RM12 4TP

Dr D Starr
The Rosewood Medical
    Centre
1 Rosewood Avenue
Elm Park
Hornchurch
Essex
RM12 5BU

Dr R E Farrow
The Surgery
58B Billet Lane
Hornchurch
Essex
RM11 1XY

The Surgery
23 Wingletye Lane
Hornchurch
Essex
RM11 3SU

HORSHAM

Dr J E Clarke
Park Surgery
Albion Way
Horsham
West Sussex
RH12 1BG

HOUNSLOW

Dr B S Mangat
The Surgery
5 Cecil Road
Hounslow
Middlesex
TW3 1NU

Family Doctor Unit
92 Bath Road
Hounslow
Middlesex
TW3 3EH

BA Travel Clinic
Eastchurch Road
Hatton Cross
Hounslow
Middlesex
TW6 7JR

Health Control Unit
Heathrow Airport
Terminal 3
Hounslow
Middlesex

Dr P S Garcha
The Hounslow Family
    Practice
Medical Centre
8 Pownall Gardens
Hounslow
Middlesex
TW3 1YW

British Airways Med Service
Speedbird House Medical
    Centre
Heathrow Airport
Hounslow
Middlesex
TW6 2JA

British Airways Medical
    Service
Queen's Building
Heathrow Airport
Hounslow
Middx
TW6 2BX

Queen's Building Medical
    Centre
Heathrow Airport Limited
Heathrow Airport
Hounslow
Middlesex
TW6 1JH

YFVC Medical Department
British Airways Medical
    Service
Building 133
PO Box 10
Hounslow
Middlesex

British Airways Travel Clinic
Eastchurch Road
Hatton Cross
Hounslow
Middlesex
TW6 2JR

Health Control Unit
Heathrow Airport
Terminal 3
Hounslow
Middlesex
TW6 1MB

Dr G M Stewart
Heathrow Airport
Terminal 3 Arrivals
Hounslow
Middlesex
TW6 1MB

HOVE

The Manor Laboratory
26 New Church Road
Hove
Sussex
BN3 4FH

The Surgery
Goodwood Court
52/54 Cromwell Road
Hove
Sussex
BN3 3DX

HOYLAKE

Dr M Burgess
Hoylake and Heols Medical
    Centre
53 Birkenhead Road
Hoylake
Wirral
L47 5AF

HUDDERSFIELD

Fieldhead Surgery
Fieldhead
Leymoor Road
Huddersfield
West Yorkshire
HD7 4QQ

The Health Centre
Commercial Road
Skelmanthorpe
Huddersfield
West Yorkshire
HD8 9DA

Dr G Eales
The Surgery
Northgate
Almondbury
Huddersfield
West Yorkshire
HD5 8RX

Dr J F W Priestman
The Health Services Centre
Shelley Lane
Kirkburton
Huddersfield
West Yorkshire
HD8 0SL

Dr M D Hopper
The Waterloo Practice
617 Wakefield Road
Waterloo
Huddersfield
HD5 9XP

HULL

Dr K J Kutte
The Surgery
415 Beverley Road
Kingston-upon-Hull
Hull
Humberside
HU5 1LX

University Health Service
University of Hull
187 Cottingham Road
Kingston-upon-Hull
Hull
Humberside
HU5 2EG

Dr N A M Somerville
The Sydenham House Group
    Practice
Boulevard
Hull
Humberside
HU3 2TA

The Central Clinic
74 Beverley Road
Kingston-upon-Hull
Hull
Humberside
HU3 1YD

Medicos Ltd Medicos House
74 Beverley Road
Kingston-upon-Hull
Hull
Humberside
HU3 1XR

Health Centre
Marmaduke Street
Heggle Road
Hull
Humberside
HU3 3BH

HUNSTANTON

Dr P E Burgess
The Surgery
9 Belgrave Avenue
Hunstanton
Norfolk
PE36 6DQ

HUNTINGDON

Dr R B Allan
Priory Field Surgery
Nursery Road
Huntingdon
Cambridgeshire
PE18 6RJ

Dr D A Haslam
The Health Centre
Whytefield Road
Ramsey
Huntingdon
Cambs
PE17 1AQ

Dr D J Martin
Parkhall Surgery
2C Parkhall Road
Somersham
Huntingdon
Cambridgeshire
PE17 3EU

HUTHWAITE

Dr E Ulliott
The Health Centre
New Street
Huthwaite
Nottinghamshire
VG17 2LR

HYDE

Dr P Bennett
Clarendon House
Clarendon Street
Hyde
Cheshire
SK14 2AG

Dr S A Barton
Hattersley Health Centre
Hattersley Road East
Hattersley
Hyde
SK14 3EH

ILFORD

The Surgery
150 Longwood Gardens
Clayhall
Ilford
Essex
IGE OBE

The Roding Hospital
Roding Lane South
Ilford
Essex
IG4 5PS

Dr J D DESAI
The Surgery
69 Belmont Road
Ilford
Essex
IG1 1YW

ILFRACOMBE

The Medical Centre
St Brannocks Road
Ilfracombe
Devon
EX34 8EG

ILLINGWORTH

Dr K S Aiyappa
Keighley Road Surgery
Illingworth
Halifax
HX2 9LL

IMMINGHAM

Dr R S P Singh
Craikhill Surgery
Immingham
South Humberside
DN40 1LP

IMPINGTON

Dr Aiden Challen
BUPA Cambs Lea Hospital
30 New Road
Impington
Cambridgeshire
CB4 4EL

IPSWICH

Orchard Street Health Centre
Ipswich
Suffolk
1P4 2PV

ISLEWORTH

The Surgery
215 Springgrove Road
Isleworth
Middlesex
TW7 4AF

ISLES OF SCILLY

Dr A J Davis
The Health Centre
St Mary's
Isles of Scilly
Cornwall
TR21 OLE

IVER

Medical Department
Pinewood Studios
Pinewood Road
Iver
Buckinghamshire
SLO ONH

ST IVES

Dr D J Rogers
Old Grammar School Surgery
1 Ramsey Road
St Ives
Huntingdon
Cambs
PE17 4BZ

IVYBRIDGE

The Ivybridge Health Centre
Station Road
Ivybridge
Devon
PL21 OAB

KEARSLEY

Dr B V Harris
Kearsley Medical Centre
Jackson Street
Kearsley
Manchester
BL4 8EP

KEIGHLEY

Dr A R Cadamy
Health Centre
Holme Lane
Cross Hills
Keighley
Yorkshire
BD20 7LG

Dr P L Dinnen
The Health Centre
Oakworth Road
Keighley
West Yorkshire
BD21 1SA

KENDAL

Dr A Meyrick
Station House Surgery
Kental
Cumbria
LA9 6SA

Dr P W Buckler
The Marde Street Surgery
Marde Street
Kendal
Cumbria
LA9 4QE

KENTON

Dr M L Levy
32A Prestwood Avenue
Kenton
Middlesex
HA3 8JZ

KESWICK

Dr M R Turnbull
The Surgery
37 Brundholme Terrace
Keswick
Cumbria
CA12 4Wb

KETTERING

Linden Medical Centre
Linden Avenue
Kettering
Northamptonshire
NN15 7NX

KIDDERMINSTER

Dr E J C Parker
Northumberland House
    Surgery
437 Stourport Road
Kidderminster
Worcester
DY11 7BL

Dr N C Jarvie
Stanmore House Surgery
Linden Avenue
Kidderminster
Worcester
DY10 3AA

Dr M B Davies
Forest Glades Medical Centre
Bromsgrove Street
Kidderminster
Worcestershire
DY10 1PE

KIDLINGTON

Dr N Bryson
Islip Surgery
Bletchindon Road
Islip
Oxon
OX5 2TQ
Tel: 0865 71666

KINERTON

Dr J Woodward
Health Care Centre
Pinnock House
Banbury Road
Kinerton
Warwickshire
CY35 OJY

KINGSKERSWELL

Dr S Giles
Kingskerswell Health Centre
School Road
Kinerton
Warwickshire
CY35 OJY

KING'S LYNN

Dr P J Whyman
Grimston Medical Centre
Congham Road
Grimston
King's Lynn
Norfolk

Dr J Z Burgess
A T Mays Travel Clinic
102 High Street
King's Lynn
Norfolk
PE30 1BW

KINGSTON

Dr C W S Alessi
Richmond Road Medical
    Centre
95 Richmond Road
Kingston
Surrey
KT2 5BT

Dr W Russell
The Surgery
3 Upper Teddington Road
Hampton Wick
Kingston
Surrey
KT1 4DL

The Surgery
14 Fairfield South
Kingston
Surrey
KT1 2UJ

Department of Pharmacy
Kingston Hospital
Wolverton Avenue
Kingston
Surrey
KT2 7QB

KINGSTON-UPON-HULL

Area Pharmaceutical Store
Springfield House
Springfield Way Anlaby
Kingston-upon-Hull
Humberside
MU10 6RZ

KINGSWINFORD

Dr N Plant
The Surgery
Summerhill
Kingswinford
West Midlands
DY6 9JG

KNARESBOROUGH

Dr D I Jobling
21 Stockwell Road
Knaresborough
North Yorkshire
HG5 OJY

KNEBWORTH

Knebworth & Marymead
    Medical Practice
The Surgery
Station Road
Knebworth
Hertfordshire

LAKENHEATH

Dr T P Daley
The Surgery
135 High Street
Lakenheath
Suffolk
IP27 9EP

LAMBERHURST

The Surgery
Lamberhurst
Tunbridge Wells
Kent
TN3 8EX

Appendix 1

LANCASTER

Ashton Road Clinic
Lancaster
Lancashire
LA4 4RR

Cleveland Medical Lab Ltd
Lancaster & Lakeland
    Nuffield Hospital
Meadowside
Lancaster
Lancashire
LA1 3RH

Dr R Sullivan
The Health Centre
Bentham
Lancaster
Lancashire
LA2 7JP

The Surgery
1 Meadowside
Lancaster
Lancashire
LA1 3AQ

LARKFIELD

Dr T J Cantor
Thornhills Medical Group
732 London Road
Larkfield
Aylesford
Kent
ME20 6BG

LAUNCESTON

Dr D M Bafer
Launceston Medical Centre
Launceston
Cornwall

LEABROOKS

Dr C Clayton
Leabrooks Medical Centre
27 Swanwick Road
Leabrooks
Derbyshire
DE55 1LJ

LEAMINGTON SPA

Croft Medical Centre
Calder Walk
Leamington Spa
Warwickshire
CV31 1SA

Dr M Forrester
Ashton House
15 George Street
Leamington Spa
CV31 1ET

LEEDS

Halton Clinic
2 Primrose Lane
Off Selby Road
Leeds 15
West Yorkshire

Dr R G Stratchan
Sunfield Medical Centre
Sunfield Place
Stanningley
Pudsey
Leeds
LS28 6DR

Area Pharmaceutical Store
Mayfair House
Shannon Street
Leeds
Yorkshire
S9 8SS

Dr K Ravi
Medexx International
Vaccination Centre
Scorpios House
Town Street
Armley
Leeds
LS12 3HS

Dr R H Dunphy
Pinfold Surgery
Pinfold Lane
Metley
Leeds
Yorkshire
LS26 9AB

Dr G P Singh
oakwood Surgery
Gledhow Rise
Leeds
Yorkshire
LS8 4AA

Dr M J Berger
Highfield Surgery
Holtdale Approach
Leeds
Yorkshire
LS16 7ST

Dr H J McGrath
The Health Centre
Gibson Lane
Kippax
Leeds
LS25 7JN

Dr R B Welch
60 Moor Grange View
Leeds
L16 5BJ

Dr R D Gilmore
Manor Park Surgery
Bellmont Close
Leeds
Yorkshire
LS13 2UP

Windsor House Surgery
2 Corporation Street
Morley
Leeds
Yorkshire
LS27 9PX

Dr J W D Moxon
Burton Croft Surgery
5 Burton Crescent
Leeds
Yorkshire
LS6 4DN

Dr Jean Jenkins
Windsor House Surgery
2 Corporation Street
Morley
Leeds
Yorkshire

LEEK

Dr N Rowley
The Stockwell Surgery
Park Medical Centre
Ball Haye Road
Leek
Stafffordshire
ST13 6QP
Tel: 0538 399398

LEICESTER

Dr S S Bhangoo
St Peter's Health Centre
Sparkenhoe Street
Leicester
Leicestershire
LE2 OTA

The Health Centre
Countes Thorpe
Leicester
Leicestershire
LE8 3QJ

BA Travel Clinic
16 High Street
Leicester
Leicestershire
LE1 5YN

Community Health Services
Leicester Area Health
    Authority
10-12 University Road
Leicester
Leicestershire
LE1 6TP

Dr Y B Shah
6 Silverdale Drive
Thormaston
Leicester
Leicestershire
LE4 8NG

The Surgery
296 Clarendon Park Road
Leicester
Leicestershire
LE2 3G

Dr R K Hirani
The Surgery
1 Shakespear Street
Loughborough
Leicester
LE11 1QQ
Tel: 0509 268060

Dr I Cross
Student Health Service
161 Welford Road
Leicester
Leicestershire
LE2 6BF
Tel: 0533 554776

The Medical Centre
University of Technology
Loughborough
Leicester
LE11 3TU
Tel: 0509 263171

LEIGH

Health Centre
Grasmere Street
Leigh
Lancashire
WN7 1XB
Tel: 0942 673578

Dr M R B Cottrill
Brookmill Medical Centre
College Street
Leigh
Lancashire
WN7 WRB
Tel: 0942 673188

LEIGH-ON-SEA

Doctor's Clinic
335 Eastwood Road North
Leight-on-Sea
Essex
SS9 4LT
Tel: 0702 529817

LEOMINSTER

Dr J E T Stokes
The Health Centre
Westfield Walk
Leominster
Herefordshire
HR6 HHD
Tel: 0568 61414

LETCHWORTH

Birchwood Surgery
232-240 Nevells Road
Letchworth
Hertfordshire
SG6 4UB
Tel: 0462 683456

LEVEN

Dr I A Jollie
The Surgery
High Style
Leven
HU17 5WL
Tel: 0964 542155

LEWES

Dr M J Heauh
School Hill House Surgery
School Hill House
Lewes
East Sussex
BN7 2LU
Tel: 0273 474194

LEYLAND

Sister Brown
British Leyland
Spurrier Works
Medical YFVC
Leyland
Lancashire

Dr R F Catherwood
Royal Ordance Plc
Occupational Health
Wigan Road
Leyland
Lancashire
PR7 6AD

LICHFIELD

Dr L Harrington
St Chad Health Centre
Dimbles Lane
Lichfield
Staffs
WS13 7HT
Tel: 0543 258990

The Minister Practice
Greenhill Health Centre
Church Street
Lichfield
Staffordshire
WS13 6JL
Tel: 0543 416655

Dr J D James
Westgate Practice Greenhill
    Health Centre
Church Street
Lichfield
Staffordshire
WS13 6JL
Tel: 0543 416633

LIFTON

Dr M A Sparrow
The Surgery
North Road
Lifton
Devon
PL16 OEH
Tel: 0566 84788

LINCOLN

Newland Health Centre
Newland
Lincoln
Lincolnshire
LN1 1XP
Tel: 0522 532321 Ext 271

Dr G F Birch
Lindum Practice
Cabourne Avenue
Lincoln
LN2 2BT
Tel: 0522 569033

Bromhead Hospital
Nettleham Road
Lincoln
Lincolnshire
LN2 3SW
Tel: 0522 540683

Dr Chapman
Glebe House
Church Road
Saxilby
Lincoln
LN1 2H7
Tel 0522 702236

LISKEARD

The Surgery
8 Dean Street
Liskeard
Cornwall
PL14 4AQ
Tel: 0579 43133

LITTLEBOROUGH

Dr R Chew
Littleborough Health Centre
Featherstall Road
Littleborough
Lancs
OL15 8HF
Tel: 0706 378433

LITTLEHAMPTON

Dr E Gerard
Littlehampton Health Centre
The Wickton Practice
Fitzalan Road
Littlehampton
Sussex
BN17 7EB
Tel: 0903 714113

LIVERPOOL

International Vacc Clinic
Sefton Gen Hospital
Smithdown Down
Liverpool
Merseyside
L3 5QA
Tel: 051 733 4020 Ext 2202

Liverpool FHSA
1st Floor
8 Matthew Street
Liverpool
L2 6RE
Tel: 051 236 4747

School of Tropical Medicine
Pembroke Place
Liverpool
Merseyside
L3 5QA
Tel: 051 708 9393

Mersey Medical Centre
General Council of British
   Shipping
Strand Street
Pier Head
Liverpool
Merseyside
L3 1DQ
Tel: 051 236 6031

Dr H Debson
MTL Medical Services
24 Hatton Garden
Liverpool
Merseyside
L5 2QA
Tel: 051 227 1873

Dr V A Harvey
Stanley Medical Centre
Stanley Road
Liverpool
Merseyside
L5 2QA
Tel: 051 207 0126

Dr B A O'Donnell
The Surgery
15 Long Lane
Garston
Liverpool
Merseyside
L19 6PE
Tel: 051 494 1445

Dr S Pande
The Surgery
14 North View
Edgehill
Liverpool
Merseyside
L7 8TS
Tel: 051 709 3779

Dr G Beaumont
The Clinical Laboratory
   Limited
27 Rodney Street
Liverpool
L1 9EH
Tel: 051-708 6767

LONDON E & EC

Dr R Petty
The International Medical
   Centre
119 Bishopgate
London
EC2M 7TH
Tel: 071 283 0634

Dr G Bulger
The Surgery
153 Hainault Road
Leytonstone
London
E11 1DT
Tel: 081-5392513

Dr M S Glenn
St Bartholomews Medical
   College
Student Health Serv
Charterhouse Square
London
EC1M 6BQ
Tel: 071 982 6057

Dr P J Guider
Rood Lane Medical Centre
10 Rood Lane
London
EC3M 8AO
Tel: 071 283 4027

Dr T Lwin
The Surgery
343 Prince Regents Lane
London
E16 3JL
Tel: 071 511 2988

Dr G Taylor
Ecclesbourne
Warwick Terrace
Leabridge Road
London
E17 9DP
Tel: 081-539 2077

The City & Hackney Health
   District
The General Council of British
   Shipping
19-23 Prescott Street
London
E1 8BB
Tel: 071 709 9221

Chief Medical Officer
The General Council of British
   Shipping
30-33 St Mary Axe
London
EC3A 8ET
Tel: 071 283 2922

Dr A H Everington
The Surgery
94 Whitehorse Lane
London
E1 4LR
Tel: 071-790 2658

Dr D Kapoor
Grange Park Medical Centre
24 Grange Park Road
Leyton
London
E10 5EP
Tel: 081 539 7940/2542

Dr H M J Kindness
The Surgery
65 London Wall
London
EC2M 7AD
Tel: 071 638 3001

Dr (Mrs) S S Kumar
1 Larkshall Road
North Chingford
London
E4 7HS
Tel: 081 529 1298

Barbican Medical Limit
No.3 White Lyon Court
The Barbican
London
EC2Y 8EA
Tel: 071 588 3146

Dr Brackenridge & Partners
The Surgery
3 Lombard Street
London
EC3V 9AL
Tel: 071 626 6985

Dr Hugh Richards
The Surgery
4 Mitre Court Chambers
4 Old Mitre Court
Fleet Street
EC4Y 7BP
Tel: 071 353 4151

Dr Sharma
The Surgery
6 Wanstead Place
Wanstead
London
E11 2SW
Tel: 081 989 2019

Dr J A Prince
The London Hospital
Occupation Health Dept.
London
E1 1BB
Tel: 071 377 7000

City Health Care Ltd
36-44 Moorgate
London
EC2 4TH
Tel: 071 638 4988

Mildmay Mission Hospital

Hackney Road
London
E2 7NA
Tel: 071 739 2331

Dr Gill & Partners
The Surgery
23 Lawrence Lane
London
EC2C 8DA
Tel: 071 606 6159

Dr P J Guider
The City Medical Centre
17 St Helens Place
London
EC3A 6DE
Tel: 071 588 6503

Dr J Richardson
Island Health
ASDA Superstore
East Ferry Road
London
E14 9BQ
Tel: 071 537 2311

Dr R K Gupta
Higman Hill Surgery
258-260 Higham High Road
Walthamstow
London
E17 5RQ
Tel: 081 527 2677

BA Travel Clinic
101 Cheapside
London
EC2V 6DT
Tel: 071 606 2977

Dr Harris-Jones
4 Snow Hill
London
EC1A 3DH
Tel: 071 236 2832

Dr M S Duggal
Healy Medical Centre
200 Upper Clapton Road
London
E5 9DH
Tel: 081 8061550/1928/1611

Dr I D Baron
237 Campbell Road
Bow
London
E3 4DP
Tel: 071 987 7555

Dr D Kelly
5 London Wall Buildings
Finsbury Circus
London
EC2M 5NT
Tel: 071 382 9989

The Medical Department
Unilever House
Blackfriars Embankment
London
EC4 4BQ
Tel: 071 822 6047

Dr R B Shah
103-105 Grove Road
Walthamstow
London
E17 8UB
Tel: 081 521 2221

Dr S A Wood
The Surgery
140 Claremont Road
Forest Gate
London
E7 0PX
Tel: 081 472 1239

London W & WC

Dr S Hunt
The Surgery
95 Burlington Lane
London
W4 3ET
Tel: 081-7471549

Dr M Scurr
The Surgery
14 Ladbrooke Gardens
London
W11 2PT
Tel: 071 792 8060

Dr D Forecast
Executive Health Centre
48 Harley Street
London
W1N 1AD
Tel: 071 323 9292

Dr A Walden
The Surgery
1 Florence Street
London
W5 3TU
Tel: 081 567 2111

Dr A Saujahi
156 Horn Lane
Acton
London
W3 6PH
Tel: 081 992 4722

Dr W M Styles
The Grove Health Centre
Goldhawk Road
London
W12 8EJ
Tel: 081 743 7153

Dr Judith Brett
Central Institutioos Health
    Service
University of London
20 Gower Street
London
WC1E 6DP
Tel: 071-6367628

Dr Helen M Murphy
The Surgery
2 Hanway Place
London
W1P 9DF
Tel: 071 323 0760

Dr M Johnson
The Surgery
11 Dundee House
145 Maida Vale
London
W9 1QP
Tel: 071 286 8566

Appendix 1

Dr A D Lauder
The Surgery
10 Corfton Road
Ealing
London
W5 2HS
Tel: 081 997 4215

Dr A M Weber
Southfield Medical Centre
89 Southfield Road
Chiswick
London
W4 1BB
Tel: 081 994 3099

Dr J S Dua
32 Elsham Road
London
W14 8HB
Tel: 071 603 5206

Dr C R Calman
The Surgery
73 Holland Park
London
W11 3SL
Tel: 071 221 4334

Dr S M Spencer
Hillcrest Surgery
337 Uxbridge Road
Acton
London
W3 9RA
Tel: 081 993 0922

Dr A Steele
Colville Health Centre
51 Kensington Park Road
London
W11 1PA
Tel: 071 727 5800

Dr C J Crowley
The Surgery
6 Queens Walk
Ealing
London
W5 1TO
Tel: 081 997 3041

Dr D S Cowen
The Surgery
61 Northfield Avenue
Ealing
London
W13 9QP

Dr C Elliott
Sterndale Surgery
74A Sterndale Road
London
W14 0HX
Tel: 071 602 3797

Dr P H Kaye
Acton Health Centre
35-61 Church Road
London
W3 8QE
Tel: 081 992 4062

Dr G Moses
IBM (UK) Ltd
Health Department
389 Chiswick High Road
London
W4 4AL

St Mary's Hospital
Praed Street
London
W2 1NY
Tel: 071-7256666

Dr A F R Hughes
The Princess Grace Hospital
42-52 Nottingham PLC
London
W1M 3FD
Tel: 071 935 2230/0541

Dr L Roodyn
The Surgery
7 Wimpole Street
London
Q1M 7AB
Tel: 071 323 1555

International Medical Centre
21 Upper Wimpole Street
London
W1M 7TA
Tel: 071 486 3063

Dr A J Rehman
93 Harley Street
London
W1N 1DG
Tel: 071 935 2079

The Surgery
1 Avenue Crescent
London
W3 8EW
Tel: 081-992 0530/1963

Dr S M Drage
Bedford Park Surgery
55 South Parade
Chiswick
London
W4 5LH
Tel: 071-994 0298/3333

Dr Christine Gardiner
The Surgery
1 Glebe Street
Chiswick
London
W4 2BD
Tel: 081-747 4800

Dr N A Thakran
Chiswick Health Centre
Fishers Lane
Chiswick
London
W4 1RX
Tel: 081 994 3576

Dr R Halvorsen
Holborn Medical Centre
64 Conduit Street
London
WC1N 3LW
Tel: 071-405 3541

West London Vaccinating
Centre
53 Great Cumberland Place
London
W1H 7LH
Tel: 071-262 6456

Pharmacy Department
Hammersmith Hospital
Du Cane Road
London
W12 0HS
Tel: 081 740 3063

Mr M D Hughes
BUPA Hospital
Dolphyn Court
Great Turnstile
Lincoln's Inn Fields
London
WC1V 7JU

Dr R Hart
The Surgery
4 Norfolk Place
London
W2 1QN
Tel: 071 723 7891

Dr R NG
British Airways Travel Clinic
9 Little Newport Street
London
WC2H 7JJ
Tel: 071-8315333

Dr P J Pettifer
Colville Health Centre
51 Kensington Park Road
London
W11 1PH
Tel: 071 727 4592

Civil Aviation House
45-49 Kingsway
London
WC2B 6TE
Tel: 071-3797311

Allied Medical Diagnostic
Clinic
21H Devonshire Place
London
W1N 1PD
Tel: 071 486 7379/7344

Dr K Kyei-Mensah
Suite 2
Lister House
11/12 Wimpole Street
London
W1M 2AB
Tel: 071 637 4805

Dr D L Cowan
YFVC
22 Carolyn Place
London
W2
Tel: 071-229 1671

Dr A V R Watkins
The Surgery
37 Addison Road
London
W14 8JH
Tel: 071 603 4992

Dr N Burbidge
The Surgery
2 Oxford Gardens
Chiswick
London
W4 3DW
Tel: 081-995 4396

Queen Charlotte's Maternity
Hospital
Goldhawk Road
London
W6 0XG
Tel: 081 740 3063

Dr H Mamdani
The Surgery
2 Burlington Gardens
Acton
London
W3 6BA
Tel: 081-992 0346

Dr D Russell
Mattock Lane Health Centre
78 Mattock Lane
Ealing
London
W13 9NZ
Tel: 081-997 9564

Trailfinders Travel Centre
Medical Advisory Centre
194 Kensington High Street
London
W8 7RG
Tel: 071 938 3999

Dr G Moses
The Surgery
143 Uxbridge Road
London
W12 9RD
Tel: 081-743 1511

Dr J Joseph
AMOCO Europe Incorporated
48 Wimpole Street
London
W1M 7BD
Tel: 071 486 7876

British Airways Travel Clinic
156 Regent Street
London
W1R 7HG
Tel: 071 439 9584

Thomas Cook Group Limited
45 Berkeley Street
London
W1A 1EB
Tel: 071 499 4000

Dr P J Travis
1 Eastfields Road
London
W3 0AA
Tel: 081 992 4331

Dr C Goodson-Wickes
The Surgery
8 Devonshire Place
London
W1N 1PB
Tel: 071 935 5011

British Airways Travel Clinic
PPP Immunisation Centre
99 New Cavendish Street
London
W1M 8FQ
Tel: 071 637 8941

Dr T Bolek
The London Medical Centre
144 Harley Street
London
W1N 1AH
Tel: 071 935!0023

Dr M Seear
The Surgery
86 Harley Street
London
W1
Tel: 071 580 3256
London N & NW

Dr C E Bangham
The Surgery
Cornwall House
Cornwall Avenue
London
N3 1LD
Tel: 081 346 1560

Dr F Born
98 Turnpike Lane
London
N8 OPH
Tel: 081-889 6770

Dr S Tailainatham
Brownlow Medical Centre
140-142 Brownlow Road
London
N11 2BD
Tel: 081 888 7775

Dr C Riley
Torrington Speedwell Practice
Torrington Park
London
N12 9SS
Tel: 081 445 7581

Dr V K Gupta
The Surgery
80 Hornsey Road
London
N7 7NN
Tel: 071 607 6475

Dr H J Kates
The Surgery
244 Tufnell Park Road
London
N19 5EW
Tel: 071 272 3200

Dr J P Kanodia
The Surgery
65 Downham Road
Islington
London
N1 5AH
Tel: 071 254 2299

Dr D Shah
Jaina House Surgery
66 Arnos Grove
London
N14 7AR
Tel: 081 886 4035

Dr S J Holdes
12 Cambridge Gardens
London
NW6
Tel: 071 624 2114

Dr D A Coffman
The Law Medical Group
Practice
9 Wrotesley Road
Willesden
London
N10 6UY
Tel: 081 965 8611

Dr J R Lubin
The Surgery
20 Derwent Gardens
London
N10 0QQ
Tel: 081 446 0171

Dr M K Lamba
The Surgery
61 Colindeep Lane
London
NW9 6DJ
Tel: 081 205 6798

Dr M H Goldman
The Surgery
NOMAD
314 Wellington Terrace
Turnpike Lane
London N8 0PX
Tel: 081 889 7014

Dr M H Goldman
The Surgery
19 Middleton Park
London
N20 0HT
Tel: 081 445 7128

Dr Sam Woko
Burnley Road Clinic
77 Burnley Road
London
NW10 1EE
Tel: 081-452 7680

Dr R K Babu-Narayan
331 Church Lane
London
NW9 8JD
Tel: 081 205 6262

Dr M Harris
Temple Fortune Health Centre
23 Temple Fortune Lane
London
NW11 7TE
Tel: 081 458 4431

Dr L Blumberg
Stamford Hill Group Practice
2 Egerton Road
London
N16 6UA
Tel: 081 800 1000

Dr C P Crosby
The Garden Hospital
46-55 Sunny Gardens Road
London
NW4 1RX
Tel: 081 203 0111

Dr T Rosengarten
Morris House Surgery
Waltheof Gardens
Tottenham
London
N17 7EB
Tel: 081 801 1277/8/9

Mrs C E Hunter
Central Middlesex Hospital
Acton Lane
London
NW10 7NS
Tel: 081-965 5733

Dr T Patalay
The Surgery
1 Arcadian Gardens
Bowes Park
London
N22
Tel: 081 888 2929

Dr L Mirvis
The Surgery
188 Golders Green Road
London
NW11 9AY
Tel: 081 455 7506/1907

Dr B Bannister
Coppett's Wood Hospital
Royal Free
Coppett's Road
Muswell Road
London
N10 1JB
Tel: 081 883 9792

Mr R K Mehta
Neasden Medical Centre
21 Tanfield Avenue
London
N22
Tel: 081 888 2929

Occupational Health Unit
Central Middlesex Hospital
Acton Lane
London
NW10 7NS
Tel: 081-965 5733

Dr S L Datoo
The Surgery
278 Watford Way
London
NW4 4UR
Tel: 081-203 1166/7
      081-637 0491

Dr P V Kumar
132 Stag Lane
Kingsbury
London
NW9 0QP
Tel: 081 204 0151

Dr M S Dave
Stuart Crescent Health Centre
Wood Green
London
N22 5UJ
Tel: 081-889 4311

Dr J M Sandford
Hampstead Group Practice
5 Elm Terrace
Constantine Road
London
NW3 2LL
Tel: 071 267 31811/2

BUPA Medical Centre
Webb House
210 Pentonville Road
King's Cross
London
NW1 9TA
Tel: 071-837 6484

British Airways Travel Clinic
Hospital for Tropical Diseases
4 St Pancras Way
London
NW1 0PE
Tel: 071-387 4411 Ext 136/137

Dr W Townsley
NW London Vaccination
   Centre
234 Hendon Way
Hendon
London
NW4 3NE
Tel: 081-202 7272

Ravenscroft Medical Centre
168 Holders Green Road
London
NW11 8BB
Tel: 081 455 9530

Dr S Gibson
Heathfield Surgery
Lyttleton Road
London
N2 OEE
Tel: 081-455 4068

Dr J Slesenger
39 Baronsmere Road
East Finchley
London
N2 9QD
Tel: 081 883 1458
London SE & SW

Dr H L Firth
The Surgery
21 Morden Hill
Lewisham
London
SE13 7NN
Tel: 081-469 2869

Dr A J Mitchell
Westminster & Pimlico GP
15 Denbigh Street
London
SW1V 2HF
Tel: 071 834 6969

Dr Guy O'Keefe
The Surgery
5 Paultons Square
London
SW3 5AS
Tel: 071 352 6464/5172

Dr K Nowak
The Surgery
Waterfall House
223 Tooting High Street
London
SW17 0TD
Tel: 081 672 1327

Dr C Grayson
The Health Centre
Sheen Lane
London
SW14 8LP
Tel: 081 876 4086

Dr J A Bochsler
Pasteur Primary Care Centre
13 Gipsy Hill
London
SE19 1QG
Tel: 081 670 7977

Dr S Curson
Princess Street Group Practice
2 Princess Street
Elephant & Castle
London
SE1 6JP
Tel: 071 928 0253

Dr R C Rathbone
The Surgery
2 Burbage Road
London
SE24 9HT
Tel: 071 274 6138

Dr J Harling
The Surgery
4 Collingham Gardens
London'SW5 0HW
Tel: 071 370 2453

Dr P J Bower
The Surgery
92 Balham Park Road
London
SW12 9EA
Tel: 081 767 8828

Dr M Sweeney
The Surgery
19 Cadogan Gardens
London
SW3 2RZ
Tel: 071 730 4114

Dr M M Ferries
The Surgery
4 Frobisher House
Dolphin Square
London
SW1 3LN
Tel: 071 798 8520

Dr V K Mittal
The Surgery
47 Boundaries Road
London '
SW1 8EU
Tel: 081 673 1476

Dr B M Aarons
The Surgery
4B Disraeli Road
London
SW15 2DS
Tel: 081 788 4836

Dr R Gribble
The Surgery
13 Pimlico Road
London
SW1W 8NA
Tel: 071 824 8234

Dr P Greenfield
The Church Lane Surgery
2 Church Lane
London
SW19 3NY
Tel: 081 542 1174

Dr M B McManus
The Surgery
91 Mitcham Lane
Streatham
London
SW16 6LY
Tel: 081 769 0705

Dr R Harris-Jones
Cassidy Health Centre
651A Fulham Road
London
SW6 6PX
Tel: 071 731 2511

Dr G C Provost
The Surgery
67 Vineyard Hill Road
Wimbledon
London
SW19 7JL
Tel: 081 947 2579

Dr T H D Evans
The Surgery
42 Fernhurst Road
London
SW6 7JW
Tel: 071 736 2540

Dr A G Adam
Forest Hill Road Group
    Practice
1 Forest Hill Road
London
SE22 0SQ
Tel: 081 693 2264

Dr P Wheeler
The Surgery
82 Sloane Street
London
SW1X 9PA
Tel: 071 245 9333

Dr P Lewins
Gallions Reach Health Centre
Bentham Road
London
SE28 8BE
Tel; 081 311 1010

Dr H P K Lee
Stockwell Group Practice
    Buckmaster House
Stockwell Park Estate
London
SW9 0UB
Tel: 071 274 3223
    Appointments
071 274 3225 Others

Dr J R Carruthers
Occupational Health Group
King's College Hospital
Denmark Iill
London
SE5 9RS
Tel: 071 326 3387

Dr A J Bakowska
Colliers Wood Surgery
58 High Street
Colliers Wood
London
SW19 2BY
Tel: 081 540 6303

Dr C Patel
The Surgery
25 Upper Tulse Hill
London
SW2 2SD
Tel: 081 674 7868

Dr B S Selvarajay
The Surgery
29 Wandsworth Bridge Road
London
SW6 2TA
Tel: 071 736 9341

Dr W Doa
Oorwood Surgery
491 Norwood Road
London
SE27 9NJ
Tel: 081 670 1000

Dr M R Kiln
Paxton Green Health Centre
1 Alleyn Park
London
SE21 8AV
Tel: 081 670 6692

British Airways Travel Clinic
Victoria Gatwick Terminal
Victoria Place
115 Buckingham Palace Road
London
SW1V 9SJ
Tel: 071 233 6661

Dr J M Critchley
Yellow Fever Vaccination
    Centre
63 Cornwall Gardens
London
SW7 4BJ
Tel: 071 937 5362

Dr A Nijihar
The Putney Clinic
1st Floor
30 High Street
Putney
London
SW15 1SQ
Tel: 081 780 2420

R M Rowland
Jenner Health Centre
201 Stabstead Road
London
SE23 7HU
Tel: 081 690 2231

Dr M Ashworth
Hurley Clinic
Ebenezer House
Kensington Lane
London
SE11 4HJ
Tel: 071 735 7918

Dr H McMichen
British Airways Travel Clinic
Basuto Medical Centre
29 Basuto Road
London
SW6 4BJ
Tel: 071 736 7557

Dr R K Srinivas
The Surgery
32 Sunburty Street
Woolwich
London
SE18 5LY
Tel: 081 854 0157

The Surgery
30 Chartfield Avenue
Putney
London
SW15 6HG
Tel: 071 788 6442

Dr J R Gayner
YFVC
79 Cadogan Place
London
SW1X 9RP
Tel: 071 723 5482

Drs Tudor Miles & Partners
The Surgery
35A High Street
Wimbledon
London
SW19 5BY
Tel: 081 946 4820

Dr N Shakir
Bridge Lane Health Centre
20 Bridge Lane
Battersea
London
SW11 3AD
Tel: 071 585 1499

Dr H Dewji
306 Lordship Lane
East Dulwich
London
SE22 8LY
Tel: 081 693 4704

Keats Clinic
Keats House
Guys Hospital
St Thomas' Street
London
SE1 9RT
Tel: 071-407 7600 Ext 3090

Director of Occupational
    Health 'A'
St Thomas Hospital
London
SE1 7EH
Tel: 071-928 9292

Dr P Rogers
PPP Medical Centre
Emblem House
London Bridge Hosp
27 Tooley Street
London
SE1 2PR
Tel: 071 407 3277

AMI Blackheath Hospital
40-42 Lee Terrace
Blackheath
London
SW3 9UD
Tel: 071-3187722

Dr J Boreham
Thurloe Health Centre
18 Thurloe Street
London
SW7 2SU
Tel: 071 225 1544

Dr A P Brown
Burney Street Practice
48 Burney Street
Greenwick
London
SE10 8EX
Tel: 081 858 0631

Dr H Patel
Myatts Field Health Centre
Patmos Road
London
SW9 7RX
Tel: 071 587 5300

Dr J Sprindler
Herne Hill Surgery
74 Herne Hill
London
SE24 9QP
Tel: 071 274 3314
    071 274 2860

Dr A Virji
Lister Health Centre
1 Camden Square
Peckham
London
SE15 3LW
Tel: 071 701 6291

The Surgery
105 Bellenden Road
London
SE15 4QZ
Tel: 071-639 9622

Dr A W Mills
South Lewisham Health
    Centre
50 Conisborough Crescent
London
SE6 2SS
Tel: 081-698 8921

Dr H M Freeman
The Surgery
12 Durham Road
London
SW20 0TW
Tel: 081-946 0069

Dr G Barclay
The Surgery
116 Norwood Road
London
SE24 9BB
Tel: 081 674 4623

Dr T M Chabuk
39 Lancaster Avenue
West Norwood
London
SE27 9EL
Tel: 081 670 3292

Dr G Straight
The Surgery
2A Pelham Street
London
SW7 3HU
Tel: 071-584 6511

Dr J M Critchley
The Surgery
53 Cornwall Gardens
London
SW7 4BD
Tel: 071-937 5362

Brocklebank Health Centre
249 Garratt Lane
London
SW8 4UD
Tel: 081-870 1341

Dr R Gulati
The Surgery
119 Northcote Road
London
SW11 6PW
Tel: 071-228 6762

Dr A Kirkland
The Surgery
Balmuir Gardens
Putney
London
SW15 6NG
Tel: 081 788 0818

Mr John Stewart
The Rowans Surgery
1 Windemere Road
Streatham
London
SW16 5HT
Tel: 071-764 0407/8

Dr N Vass
Winstanley Group Practice
Huitt Square Surgery
Winstanley Estate
London
SW11 2HS
Tel: 071 228 8988

Dr Hazel Richardson/Barnes
Surgery
351 Danesbury Avenue
Roehampton
London
SW15 4DU
Tel: 081 876 6666

Dr N Vass
515 Old York Road
Wandsworth
London
SW18 1TF
Tel: 081 874 6894

Dr I C Ung
56 Blairderry Road
Streatham Hill
London
SW2 4SB
Tel: 081 671 3340

Dr A M Vincent
The Surgery
11 Sloane Court West
London
SW3 4TD
Tel: 071-730 1142

Avicenna Clinic
6 Penywern Road
London
SW5 9ST
Tel: 071 373 3196/7

Cromwell Hospital
Cromwell Road
London
SW5 0TU
Tel: 071 370 4233

Dr S M Jefferies
The Surgery
292 Mucster Road
Fulham
London
SW6 6BQ
Tel: 071 385 1965

Dr R T Jenkins
The Surgesy
630 Fulham Road
London
SW6 5RS
Tel: 071 736 4344

The Surgery
82 Lillie Road
London
SW6 1TN
Tel: 071 386 9299

Dr Scurr
The Surgery
63 High Street
London
SW1V 4HR
Tel: 071 792 8060

Dr M M Ferris
5 Howard House'Dolphin
Square
London
SW1 3LN
Tel: 071 798 8520

Dr P Dorrington Ward
The Surgesy
95A Jermyn Street
London
SW1Y 6JE
Tel: 071 930 2800

Dr I C Perry
The Surgery
19 Clivedon Place
London
SW1 8HD
Tel: 071-730 8045

Dr P Greenfield
The Church Lane Surgery
2 Church Lane
London
SW19 3NY
Tel: 081 542 1174

Dr A P Brown
Burney Street Practice
48 Burney Street
Greenwich
London
SE10 8EX
Tel: 081 858 0631

Dr M R Kiln
Paxton Green Health Centre
1 Alleyn Park
London
SE21 8AV
Tel: 081 670 6692

Dr B K Sinha
2 Birchdale Road
Forest Gate
London
Tel: 081-472 1600

LONDON COLNEY

Dr N P Kedia
The Surgery
45 Kings Road
London Colney
Hertfordshire
AL2 1ES
Tel: 0727 822138

LONGFIELD

Dr N Ramanathan
The Surgery
23 Pincroft Wood
New Barn
Longfidld
Kent
DA3 7HB

LOUGHBOROUGH

Dr P D Gordon
East Leake Health Centre
Gotham Lane
East Leake
Loughborough
Leicester
LE12 67G
Tel: 0569 852181

LOUGHTON

Dr C Jenkins
Loughton Health Centre
The Drive
Loughton
Essex
1G10 1HW
Tel: 081 502 5514

LOWESTOFT

Andaman Surgery
303 Long Road
Lowestoft
Suffolk
NR33 9DF
Tel: 0502 517346

LUTTERWORTH

Dr B L Masharani
Health Centre
Gilmorton Road
Lutterworth
Leicestershire
LE17 4EB
Tel: 0455 552346

LUTON

The Surgery
163 Dunstable Road
Luton
Bedfordshire
LU1 1BW
Tel: 0582 23553/5

Liverpool Road Health Centre
Liverpool Road
Luton
Bedfordshire
LU1 1HH
Tel: 0583 31321/423302

Dr P Eroto-Critou
Medical Centre
Lucas Gardens
Barton Hilms
Luton
Bedfordshire
Tel: 0582 597737

Dr D L Stevenson
Luton and Dunstable Hospital
Occupational Health
   Department
Lewsey Road
LUTON
Bedfordshire
LU4 0DZ
Tel: 0582 491122 Ext 2066/2249

Dr S Warringer
The Surgery
26 Ashcroft Road
Stopsley
LUTON
Bedfordshire
Tel: 0582 22555

Dr J G Cochrane
The Surgery
37A Linden Road
LUTON
Bedfordshire
LU4 9OZ
Tel: 0582 572817

Dr Melville & Partners
Whitehorse Vale
Barton Hills
LUTON
Bedfordshire
LU3 4AD
Tel: 0582 490087

LYMINGTON

Dr D D Bodley Scott
The Surgery
Wistaria
St Thomas Street
Lymington
Hampshire
SO14 9ND

Chawton House Surgery
St Thomas Street
Lymington
Hampshire
SO41 9ND
Tel: 0590 672953

Dr D S Browne
The Surgery
Station Road
Sway
Lymington
Hampshire
SO41 6BA
Tel: 0590 68217

LYMM

Dr P N J Cottrill
Brookfield Surgery
Whitbarrow Road
Lymm
Cheshire
WA13 9AD
Tel: 0925 756969

MAIDSTONE

Maidstone District General
   Hospital
Hermitage Lane
Maidstone
Kent
ME16 9AP
Tel: 0622 728029

MAIDENHEAD

Claremont Surgery
2 Cookham Road
Maidenhead
Berkshire
SL6 8AJ
Tel: 0628 73033

Dr M R Patch
Cedars Surgery Wilderness F
   C
8 Cookham Road
Maidenhead
Berkshire
SL6 8AJ
Tel: 0628 20458

Dr T M Mitchell Fox
Mensana Medical
1 The Crescent
Maidenhead
Berkshire
SL6 6EL
Tel: 0628 28028

Dr P J Shaw
The Symonds Medical Centre
25 All Saints Avenue
Maidenhead
Berkshire
SL6 6EL
Tel: 0628 28028

MALMESBURY

Dr N J Pickering
Gable House Surgery
46 High Street
Malmesbury
Wiltshire
SN16 9AT
Tel: 0666 826026

MALPAS

The Surgery
Laurel Bank
Malpas
Cheshire
SY14 8PS
Tel: 0948 860205

MALTON

Dr C J Diggory
Derwent Surgery
Norton Road
Malton
North Yorkshire
YO17 0PF
Tel: 0653 600069

MALVERN

The Surgery
28A Avenue Road
Malvern
Worcestershire
WR14 3BG
Tel: 0684 574773

MANCHESTER

Monsall Hospital
Newton Heath
Manchester
M10 8WR
Tel: 061 205 2393

British Airways Travel Clinic
St Mary's Gate
19-21 Market Street
Manchester
M1 1PU
Tel: 061 832 3019

Manchester Travel Clinic
Alexandra Park Health Centre
2 Whitswood Close
Manchester
M16 7AW
Tel: 061-227 9896

The Surgery
63 Manchester Road
Swinton
Manchester
M27 1FX
Tel: 061 7944343

Manchester Airport Plc
Medical Unit Room 109
1st Floor Tower Block
Manchester Airport
Manchester
M22 5PA
Tel: 061 489 3344

Dr B Hope
Irlam Health Centre
MacDonald Road
Irlam
Manchester
M30 5LH
Tel: 061 775 5421

Dr W R Fraser
154 Church Road
Urmston
Manchester
M31 1DJ
Tel: 061 748 5665

Dr I G Donnan
MSF Aviation Ltd
Manchester Airport
(South Side)
Wilmslow
Cheshire
SK9 4LL
Tel: 061 4991444

Dr M K Montrose
Hollyhedge Surgery
283 Hollyhedge Road
Crossacres
Manchester
M22 4QR
Tel: 061 4289411

University of Manchester
Occupational Health Service
William Kay House
327 Oxford Street
Manchester
M13 9PG
Tel: 061 275 6971

Dr P W Thomas
Redbank Health Centre
Unsworth Street
Radcliffe
Manchester
M26 0GA
Tel: 061 723 4028

Pharmacy Department
North Manchester General
  Hospital
Delaunays Road
Crumpsall
Manchester
M8 6RB
Tel: 061-795 4567

Dr D P Singh
The Surgery
417 Chorley Road
Swinton
Manchester
M27 3AQ
Tel: 061 7944239

Dr P M Sankey
Windward Group Practice
68 Worsley Road
Manchester
M28 4SN
Tel: 061 794 1603/4

Dr A S Finke
Colleigate Medical Centre
Brideoak Street
Manchester
M8 7AX
Tel: 061 205 4364

Dr S L Goodman
Ladybarn Group Practice
177 Mauldeth Road
Fallowfiemd
Manchester
M14 6CE

Dr P A Dixon
The Surgery
53-55 Crescent Road
Crumsall
Manchester
M8 7JT
Tel: 061 740 2213

MANSFIELD

Dr E S Steiner
Roundwood Surgery
Wood Street
Mansfield
NG18 1QQ
Tel: 0623 648880

MARCHWOOD

Dr S Hill-Cousins
The Surgery
Old Malthouse
Main Road
Marchwood
Southampton
SO4 4HS
Tel: 0703 871233

MARGATE

Northdown Surgery
St Antony's Way
Cliftonville
Margate
Kent
CT9 2TR
Tel: 0843 296413

Dr B Summerfield
The Limes Surgery
Hawley Street
Margate
CT9 1PU
Tel: 0843 227567

MARKET DEEPING

Dr S P Hughes
The Health Centre
Douglas Road
Market Deeping
Peterborough
PE6 8BA
Tel: 0778 342 388

MARKET DRAYTON

Dr Alan Bremner
Draylon Medical Practices
Cheshire Street
Market Drayton
Shropshire
TF9 3BS
Tel: 0630 652158

MARLBOROUGH

The Surgery
High Street
Ramsbury
Marlborough
Wilts
SN8 2QT
Tel: 0672 20366

The Surgery
Burbage
Marlborough
Wilts
SN8 3TA
Tel: 0672 810566

Drs Spink & Partners
The Doctors House
Victoria Road
Marlow
Buckinghamshire
SL7 1DN
Tel: 0628 4666/9

MATLOCK

Dr MacFarlane
The Practice
8 Imperial Road
Matlock
Derbyshire
DE4 3NL
Tel: 0629 582461

The Surgery
Roseleigh
9 Lime Grove Walk
Matlock
Derbyshire
DE4 3FD
Tel: 0629 583223

Dr R A P Curtis
The Surgery
Matlock Clinic
Lime Grove Walk
Matlock
Derbyshire
DE4 3FD
Tel: 0629 582107

Dr D M Clark
The Medical Centre
Two Dales
Marlock
Derbyshire
Tel: 0629 733205

MELKSHAM

Dr S A Rosser
Giffords Surgery
Lowbourne
Melksham
Wiltshire
SN12 7EA
Tel: 0225 703370

MELTON MOWBRAY

Dr H Hollis
Latham House Medical
   Practice
Sage Cross Street
Melton Mowbray
Leicestershire
LE13 1NX
Tel: 0664 60406

MEOPHAM

Dr N Benn
Meopham Medical Centre
Wrotham Road
Mempham
Kent
DA13 0AH
Tel: 0474 814068

MIDDLESBROUGH

West Lane Hospital
Acklam Road
Middlesbrough
Cleveland
TS5 4EE
Tel: 813144 Ext: 265

Dr A Cuthbert
Martonside Medical Centre
1A Martonside Way
Middlesbrough
Cleveland
TS4 3BV
Tel: 0642 812266

Dr N T Rowell
The Health Centre
Middlesbrough
Cleveland
TS1 2NX
Tel: 0642 242192

Occupational H/C Ltd
Whalley Drive
Bletchley
Milton Keynes
Buckinghamshire
MK3 6EN
Tel: 0908 75194/5

MITCHAM

Dr G Hollier
62 Manor Road
Mitcham
Surrey
CR4 1JB
Tel: 081 764 2666

MORETON-IN-MARSH

Dr P S Lutter
White House Surgery
High Street
Moreton-in-Marsh
GL56 0AT
Tel: 0608 501317

Dr R J Birts
Mann Cottage
Moreton-in-Marsh
Gloucestershire
GL56 OLA
Tel: 0608 50764

MORPETH

Dr T B Scott
Greystoke Surgery
Kings Avenue
Morpeth
Northumberland
NE61 1JA
Tel: 0670 511398

Appendix 1

Dr John Lalor
The Surgery
Scots Gap
Morpeth
Northumberland
NE18 0PF
Tel: 0670 74216

Dr C Marr
Howard Road Medical Group
6 Howard Road
Morpeth
Northumberland
NE61 1JE
Tel: 0670 517300

MORTIMER

Dr I L C Bray
The Surgery
Mortimer
Berkshire
RG7 3SQ
Tel: 0734 332436

MUCH HADHAM

Much Hadham Health Centre
Ash Meadow
Much Hadham
Herts
SG10 6DE
Tel: 0279 842243

NEEDHAM MARKET

Dr M Watson
The Surgery
33 High Street
Needham Market
Suffolk
IP6 8AL
Tel: 0442 720666

NELSON

Dr P K Guha
Surgery 3
The Health Centre
Leeds Road
Nelson
Lancashire
BB9 9TJ
Tel: 0282 698036

NEWARK

The Surgery
Lomnard Street
Newark
Nottingham
Nottinghamshire
NG24 1XG
Tel: 0636 702363

Dr J Dennis
The Medical Centre
Collingham
Newark
Nottinghamshire
NG23 7LB
Tel: 0636 892156

Dr V R Twyman
The Health Centre
50 Barnby Gate
Newark
Nottinghamshire
NG24 1QD
Tel: 0636 704226

Dr A D Garrow
The Fountain Medical Centre
Sherwood Avenue
Newark
NG24 1QH
Tel: 0636 704378

NEW BARNET

Dr Thomas
The Surgery
46 Station Road
New Barnet
Herts
EN5 1QH
Tel: 081 441 4425

NEWBURY

The Health Centre
Thatcham
Newbury
Berkshire
RG13 4HH
Tel: 0635 67171

Dr P F Sievers
The Surgery
St Mary's Road
Newbury
Berkshire
RG13 1ES
Tel: 0635 31444

NEWCASTLE-UNDER-LYME

Miller Street Surgery
1 Miller Streeu
Newcastle-Under-Lyme
Staffordshire
ST5 1JD
Tel: 0782 711618

Dr Latif M Hussain
The Surgery
123 Liverpool Road
Cross Heath
Newcastle-Under-Lyme
Staffordshire
ST5 9ER
Tel: 0782 637082

Dr D G Garvie
Wolstanton Medical Centre
Palmerston Street
Newcastle-Under-Lyme
Staffordshire
ST5 8QN
Tel: 0782 627403

Dr M S Smith
19B Hanover Street
Newcastle-Under-Lyme
Staffordshire
ST5 1EN
Tel: 0782 615367

NEWCASTLE-UPON-TYNE

Dr R Brantingham
The Saville Medical Group
5 Saville Place
Newcastle-Upon-Tyne
NE1 8DQ
Tel: 091 232 4274

Conrad & Rye
5 Osborne Avenue
Jesmond
Newcastle-Upon-Tyne
NE2 1PQ
Tel: 091 281 0041

Graingerville Clinic
4 Graingerville North
Westgate Road
Newcastle-Upon-Tyne
Tel: 091 273 9560

Dr A J N May
The Health Centre
Thornhill Road
Ponteland
Newcastle-Upon-Tyne
NE20 9PZ
Tel: 0661 25513

Dr M A Bortwick
The Surgery
200 Osborne Road
Jesmond
Newcastle-Upon-Tyne
NE2 3LD
Tel: 091 281 4777

NEWHAVEN

Newhaven Health Centre
Chapel Street
Newhaven
East Sussex
BN9 9PN
Tel: 0273 516066

NEWMARKET

Dr K Sriskandan
The Rookery Medical Centre
Newmarket
Suffolk
CB8 8NW

NEW MALDEN

The Surgery
72 Commbe Road
New Maldon
Surrey
Tel: 081 949 4422

Dr J A Barratt
229 West Barnes Lane
New Maldon
Surrey
KT3 6JD
Tel: 081 336 1773

NEWPORT

Dr Snead
Wellington Road Surgery
Newport
Shropshire
TF10 7HG
Tel: 0952 811677

NEWPORT (ISLE OF WIGHT)

St Mary's Hospital
Newport
Isle of Wight
Tel: 0983 524081 Ext: 4202

NEWPORT PAGNELL

The Health Centre
British Airways Travel Clinic
Newport Pagnell
Buckinghamshire
MK16 8EA
Tel: 0908 611767

Dr A C Paton
The Kingfisher Surgery
Elthorne Way
Newport Pagnell
Buckinghamshire
MK19 0JR
Tel: 0908 618265

NEWICK

Dr P G Estcourt
The Health Centre
Newick
Lewes
East Sussex
BN8 4LR
Tel: 0825 722272

NEWQUAY

Dr S A Brown
The Health Centre
St Thomas Road
Newquay
Cornwall
TR7 1RS
Tel: 0637 873921

Dr E J Holland
The Health Care Centre
30/32 Trebarwith Crescent
Newquay
Cornwall
TR7 1BX
Tel: 0637 874434

NORMANTON

Dr D Brown
Princess Street Surgery
Normanton
West Yorkshire
WF6 1AB
Tel: 0924 892480

NORTHALLERTON

Dr D J Dickson
The Surgery, Mowbray House
277 North End
Northallerton
North Yorkshire
DL7 8DP
Tel: 0609 775281

NORTHAMPTON

Dr A Sutton
16 London Road
Roade
Northampton
Northants
NN7 2NN
Tel: 0604 863100

The Clinic
67 St Giles Street
Northampton
NN1 5DQ
Tel: 0604 37221 Ext 2315

Northampton Area Health
Authority
St Edmunds Hospital
Clare House
Wellingborough Road
Northants
NN1 3QS

Dr P B Medcalf
Abington Medical Centre
Beech Avenue
Northampton
Northants
NN3 2JG
Tel: 0604 791999

NORTHFLEET

Dr P J Mitchell
The Surgery
The Shrubbery
65A Perry Street
Northfleet
Kent
DA11 8RD
Tel: 0474 356661

Dr A Morgan
Granby Place Surgery
1 High Street
Northfleet
Kent
DA11 9EY
Tel: 0474 352447

Dr J S Carlisle
The Surgery
34 Fairview Road
Istead Place
Northfleet
Kent
DA13 9Dr
Tel: 0474 355331

NORTH MYMMS

Dr J Whiteley
Potterels Medical Centre
Station Road
North Mymms
Hertfordshire
AL9 7SN
Tel: 0707 273339

NORTH SHIELDS

Dr G D Thomson
The Health Centre
Spring Terrace
North Shields
Tyne and Wear
NE29 0HQ
Tel: 091 296 1588

NORTH WALSHAM

Dr D Pikersgill
Birchwood Medical Practice
Park Lane
North Walsham
Norfolk
NR28 0BQ
Tel: 0692 402035

NORTHWICH

Dr A M Rossall
Danesbridge Medical Centre
London Road
Northwich
Cheshire
CW9 5HR
Tel: 0606 49145

Dr J M Torrance
The Surgery
5 Darwin Street
Northwich
Cheshire
CW8 1BU
Tel: 0606 74863

Dr R J Murphy
Witton Street Surgery
162 Witton Street
Northwich
Cheshire
CW9 5QY
Tel: 0606 45261

NORTHWOOD

Dr S Shackman
The Surgery
Mount Vernon Surgery
Rickmansworth Road
Northwood
Middlesex
Tel: 09274 28488

NORWICH

Dr P G Manson-Bahr
The Health Centre
Long Stratton
Norwich
Norfolk
NR3 3DL
Tel: 0603 30333

British Airways Travel Clinic
Oak Street Medical Practice
Norwich
Norfolk
NR3 3DL
Tel: 0603 765209

The Health Centre
West Pottergate
Norwich
Norfolk
NR2 4BX
Tel: 0603 620263

Stores Section, Pharmacy
Dept
Norfolk and Norwich
Hospital
Wesses Street
Norwich
Norfolk
Tel: 0603 28377

University of East Anglia
Health Centre
Norwich
Norfolk
NR4 7TJ
Tel: 0603 592172

NOTTINGHAM

Dr C A Brown
The Manor Surgery
Middle Street
Beeston
Nottingham
NR9 1GA
Tel: 0602 256127

Meadows Health Centre
1 Bridgeway Centre
The Meadows
Nottingham
NG2 2JG
Tel: 0602 415333 Ext 209

The Calverton Practice
St Wimfrid Square
Calverton
Nottingham
NG14 6FP
Tel: 0602 653302

BA Travel Centre
Victoria Health Centre
Glasshouse Street
Nottingham
NG1 3LW
Tel: 0602 504058

Dr P Lavelle
John Ryle Health Centre
Clifton Estate
Nottingham
NG11 8EW
Tel: 0602 212970

Dr A Wood
Keyworth Health Centre
Bunny Lane
Keyworth
Nottingham
NG12 5JU
Tel: 0602 3527

Dr J S McCraken
The Surgery
Church Close
Rise Park
Nottingham
NG5 5EB
Tel: 0602 272525

Dr P W F Lane
The Health Centre
Midland Street
Nottingham
NG10 1NY
Tel: 0602 732157

OLD AMERSHAM

Dr B L Neal
Rectory Meadow Surgery
School Lane
Old Amersham
Buckinghamshire
HP7 0HG
Tel: 0494 72771

OLDHAM

Dr M A Johnson
The Clinic
Smithy Lane
Uppermill
Nr Oldham
Lancashire
OLD3 6AH
Tel: 0457 872228

Dr J H Rice
The Glodwick
Glodwick Road
Oldham
Lancashire
OL4 1YN
Tel: 061 652 5311

Dr M G Boden
Chadderton Town Health
Centre
Middleton Road
Chadderton
Oldham
OL9 0LH
Tel: 061 652 5432

ORMSKIRK

Dr S P Frampton
18 Derby Street
Ormskirk
Lancashire
L39 2BY
Tel: 0695 579501

ORPINGTON

Dr J M R Campbell
Occupational Health
    Department
Farnborough Hospital
Orpington
Kent
BR6 8ND
Tel: 0689 853333 Ext 467/379

Dr J Brennan
Crofton Surgery
109A Crofton Road
Orpington
Kent
BR6 8HX
Tel: 0689 878509

OSWESTRY

Willow Street Medical Centre
Oswestry
Shropshire
SY11 1AJ
Tel: 0691 653143

OTFORD

Dr David Evans
Oxford Medical Practice
Leonard Avenue
Otford
Nr Sevenoaks
Kent
TN14 5RB
Tel: 09592 3929

OXFORD

The Manor Surgery
Osler Road
Headington
Oxford
Oxfordshire
OX3 9BP
Tel: 0865 62535

North Oxford Medical Centre
96 Woodstock Road
Oxford
Oxfordshire
OX2 7NE
Tel: 0865 311005

Dr C Kenyon and Partners
19 Beaumont Street
Oxford
Oxfordshire
OX1 2NA
Tel: 0865 244688

John Radcliffe Hospital
Level 2 Brown Waiting Area
Headington
Oxford
Oxfordshire
OX2 6HE
Tel: 0865 249891 Ext 4816

Dr R Armstrong
The Jerico Health Centre
Walton Street
Oxford
Oxfordshire
OX2 6NW
Tel: 0865 311234

Dr Bent Jeul-Jensen
University of Oxford
Radcliffe Infirmary
Woodstock Road
Oxford
Oxfordshire
OX2 6HE
Tel: 0865 270079

The Health Centre
Blackbird Leys Road
Oxford
Oxfordshire
OX4 5HL
Tel: 0865 778244

Dr G Gancz
The Surgery
9 King Edward Street
Oxford
Oxfordshire
OX1 4JA
Tel: 0865 242657

Dr R Armstrong
West Oxford Health Centre
Binsey Lane
Oxford
OX2 0EX
Tel: 0865 246495

Dr G Scott
Wychwood Surgery
62 High Street
Milton-under-Wychwood
Oxford
Oxfordshire
OX7 6LE
Tel: 0993 831061

St Bartholomew's Medical
    Centre
Manzil Way
Cowley Road
Oxford
Oxfordshire
OX4 1XB
Tel: 0865 242334

Dr S A K S Verjee
Kennington Health Centre
200 Kennington Road
Kennington
Oxford
Oxfordshire
OX1 5PY
Tel: 0865 730911

Jericho Health Centre
Walton Street
Oxford
OX2 6NW
Tel: 0865 59993

Dr D W Thurston
Donnington Health Centre
1 Henley Avenue
Oxford
OX1 4DH
Tel: 0865 774844

OXSHOTT

Dr R Draper
Oxshott Medical Practice
The Village Centre
Holtswood Road
Oxshott
Surrey
KT22 0QL
Tel: 0372 844000

PAIGNTON

The Clinic
Midvale Road
Paignton
Devon
TQ4 5BD
Tel: 0803 522762

Dr E Southall
Mayfield Medical Centre
37 Totnes Road
Paignton
Devon
TQ4 5LA
Tel: 0803 558257

PAR (CORNWALL)

Dr B Hannett
Middleway Surgery
St Blazey
Par
Cornwall
PL24 2JL
Tel: 072681 2019

PENZANCE

Health Clinic
Bellair
Alverton
Penzance
Cornwall
TR18 4TA
Tel: 0736 62321

Dr M H Long
Penalverne Surgery
Penzance
Cornwall
TR18 2RE
Tel: 0736 63361

Dr M Hersant
Sunnyside Surgery
Hawkins Road
Penzance
Cornwall
TR18 4LT
Tel: 0736 63340

Dr R R Dyke
Alverton Surgery
7 Alverton Terrace
Penzance
Cornwall
TR18 4JH
Tel: 0736 63191

PENSHURST

Dr E M J Law
The Surgery
Penshurst
Kent
TN11 8BP
Tel: 870208

PERSHORE

The Health Centre
Priest Lane
Pershore
Worcestershire
WR10 1Dr
Tel: 0386 552424

PETERBOROUGH

Jenner Health Centre
Whittlesey
Peterborough
Cambridgeshire
PE7 4EJ
Tel: 0733 203601

Yaxley Group Practice Health
    Centre
Landsdowne Road
Yaxley
Peterborough
Cambridgeshire
PE7 3JL
Tel: 0733 240478

Dr L Jacobs
1 North Street
Peterborough
Cambridgeshire
PE1 2RA
Tel: 0733 312525

Dr R C Patel
Werrington Health Centre
13 Skaters Way
Werrington
Peterborough
Cambridgeshire
PE4 6DG
Tel: 0733 78231

Dr A E Price
Screening Department
Fitzwilliam Hospital
Milton Way
South Bretton
Peterborough
Cambridgeshire
PE3 8YQ
Tel: 0733 261717 Ext 2323

PETERSFIELD

Dr D J Wilders
The Spain Surgery
28 The Spain
Petersfield
Hampshire
GU32 3LA
Tel: 0730 68585

PETWORTH

Dr Simon Pett
The Surgery
Petworth
West Sussex
GU28 0LP
Tel: 0798 42248

PEWSEY

Dr P D Jenkins
The Surgery
Upavon
Pewsey
Wiltshire
SN9 6DZ
Tel: 0980 630221

PICKERING

Dr T J Thornton
The Ropery
Pickering
North Yorkshire
YO18 8DY
Tel: 0751 72441

PINNER

Dr A S Kelshiker
The Pinner Medical Centre
8 Eastcote Road
Pinner
Middlesex
HA5 1HF
Tel: 081 866 5766

PLYMOUTH

Community Health
    Department
Scott Hospital
Beacon Park Road
Plymouth
Devon
PL2 2PQ

Dr M W Calder
Beaumont Villa Surgery
23 Beaumont Road
St Judes
Plymouth
PL4 9BL
Tel: 0752 669535

Dr R Hirst
The Health Centre
Yealmpton
Plymouth
Devon
PL8 2EA
Tel: 0752 880567

Dr S W Millard
Plympton Health Centre
Mudge Way
Plympton
Plymouth
PL7 3PS
Tel: 0752 348884

Appendix 1

Dr C E Wilson
Plympton Health Centre
Plympton
Plymouth
PL7 3PS
Tel: 0752 341474

Dr C P Fletcher
Woolwell Medical Centre
School Drive
Woolwell
Plymouth
Devon
PL6 7TH
Tel: 0752 695299

PONTEFRACT

Dr R K Aggarnal
The White Rose Surgery
Exchange Street
South Elmsall
Pontefract
West Yorkshire
WF9 2RD
Tel: 0977 642412

Dr W J Belk
College Lane Surgery
Bamsley Road
Ackworth
Pontefract
West Yorkshire
WF7 7HZ
Tel: 0977 611023

Dr Chandy
The Surgery
69 Stockingate
South Kirby
Pontefract
West Yorkshire
WF9 3SE
Tel: 0977 642252

Fairwood Surgery
Carleton Glen
Pontefract
West Yorkshire
WF8 1SJ
Tel: 0977 703235

POOLE

Dr J S C Scott
Carlisle House
53 Lagland Street
Poole
Dorset
BH15 1QD
Tel: 0202 678484

Dr D Williams
3 Parkstone Road
Poole
Dorset
BH15 2NN
Tel: 0202 676461

Dr G Oktekin
Birchwood Medical Centre
Northmead Drive
Creekmoor
Poole
Dorset
BH17 7XW
Tel: 0202 697639

Dr D Dent
Heatherview Medical Centre
2 Alder Park
Alder Road
Poole
Dorset
BH12 4AY
Tel: 0202 743678

Dr D P Muir
9 Mitchell Road
Canford Heath
Poole
Dorset
BH17 7UE
Tel: 0202 672474

PORT ISAAC

Dr J L Lunny
The Surgery
Hillson Close
Port Isaac
Cornwall
PL29 3TR
Tel: 0208 880222

PORTSMOUTH

Battenburg Avenue Clinic
North End
Portsmouth
Hampshire
PO2 0TA
Tel: 0705 664235

Dr B N Russell
The Drayton Surgery
274 Havant Road
Drayton
Portsmouth
Hampshire
PO6 1PA
Tel: 0705 370422

The Surgery
25 Osborne Road
Southsea
Portsmouth
Hants
PO5 3ND
Tel: 0705 821371

The Surgery
23 Landport Terrace
Southsea
Portsmouth
Hants
PO1 2RG
Tel: 0705 736006

POTTERS BAR

Parkfield Medical Centre
The Walk
Potters Bar
Hertfordshire
EN6 1QH
Tel: 0707 59923

POULTON-LE-FYLDE

Dr M J Evans
Queensway Surgery
Poulton-Le-Fylde
Blackpool
Lancashire
FY6 7ST
Tel: 0253 890219

POYNTON

Dr M Gradwell
Priorsleigh Group Practice
24 London Road North
Poynton
Cheshire
SK12 1RA
Tel: 0625 872299

PRESCOT

Mr A C Baker
Whiston Hospital
Pharmacy Department
Warrington Road
Prescot
Lancashire
L35 5Dr

PRESTON

The Surgery
4 The Drive
Longton
Preston
Lancashire
PR4 5AJ
Tel: 0772 613123

Appendix 1

Dr R Hodkinson
Stonebridge Surgery
Preston Road
Longridge
Preston
Lancashire
PR3 3AP
Tel: 0772 783271

British Aerospace Aircraft
    Group
Warton Aerodrome
Warton
Preston
Lancashire
PR4 1AX
Tel: 0772 633333

Dr N G Saha
The Surgery
310 St Georges Road
Deepdale
Preston
Lancashire
PR2 4PR
Tel: 0772 54546

Dr S Chori
The Surgery
104 Woodplumpton Road
Fulwood
Preston
PR2 2LR
Tel: 0772 729756

PRESTWICH

Dr J Schryer
Whittaker Lane Medical
    Centre
Whittaker Lane
Prestwich
M25 5EX
Tel: 061 7731580

PRINCES RISCOROUGH

The Surgery
Wellington House
Aylesbury Road
Princes Risborough
Buckinghamshire
HP17 0AX
Tel: 08444 4488

PRUDHOE

Dr S J Quilliam
The Castle Surgery
Kepwell Bank Top
Prudhoe
Northumberland
NE42 3PW
Tel: 0661 832209

PUDSEY

Dr R J Ross
Pudsey Health Centre
18 Millberry Street
Pudsey
LS28 7XP
Tel: 570711

PURLEY

BA Travel Clinic
Claremont House
2 Woodcote Valley Road
Purley
Surrey
CR2 3AC
Uel: 081-668 0801

RADMETT

The Red House
124 Watling Street
Radlett
Hertfordshire
WD7 8HB
Tel: 0923-855606

Shenley Hospital
Shenley
Radlett
Hertfordshire
WD7 9HB
Tel: 0923-765631

Radlett Health Centre
8 Letchmore Road
Radlett
Hertfordshire
WD7 8HT
Tel: 0923-856017

RAINHAM

Dr I R Hamirani
The Health Centre
39 Mungo Park Road
Rainham
Essex
RM12 7PB
Tel: 04027-54797

RAMSGATE

Dr P Attwood
The Surgery
Wideham Avenue
Ramsgate
Kent
CT1 8AY
Tel: 0843-593420

Dr J D Beale
The Grange Medical Centre
Westcliffe Road
Ramsgate
Kent
CT11 9LJ
Tel: 0843-595051

RAYLEIGH

Dr G P Kittle
Church View Surgery
Burley House
15-17 High Street
Rayleigh
Essex
SS6 7DY
Tel: 0268-774477

READING

British Airways Travel Clinic
Chancellor House
6 Shinfield Road
Reading
Berkshire
RG2 7BW
Tel: 0734-311696

Goring & Woodgate Medical
    Practice
Redcross Road Surgery
Goring
Reading
Berkshire
RG8 9HG
Tel: 0491-872372

The Surgery
41 Russell Street
Reading
Berkshire
RG1 7XD
Tel: 0734-596812

The Surgery
72 Victoria road
Mortimer
Reading
Berkshire
RG7 3SQ
Tel: 0734-332436

Western Elms Surgery
317 Oxford Road
Reading
Berkshire
RG3 1AU
Tel: 0734-590257

Dr A Oldham
The Surgery
Chalfont Close
Chalfont Way
Reading
Berkshire
RG6 2HZ
Tel: 0734-755666

Dr A Churchilm
Grovelands Medical Centre
701 Oxford Road
Reading
Berkshire
RG3 1HG
Tel: 0734-560457

Dr J C Lade
The London Vale Practice
Hurricane Way
Woodley
Reading
Berkshire
RG5 4UK
Tel: 0734-691360

21 Reading Road
Pangbourne
Reading
Berkshire
RG8 7LR
Tel: 0734-842234

REDBRIDGE

The Roding Hospital
Roding Lane South
Redbridge
Essex
IG4 5PZ
Tel: 081-551 1100

REDDITCH

Smallwood Health Centre
Church Green West
Redditch
Worcestershire
B97 4DJ
Tel: 0527-65444

The Surgery
Adelaide Street
Redditch
Worcestershire
B97 4AL

REDRUTH

The Surgery
Dargai House
Allexandra Road
Illogan
Redruth
Cornwall
TR16 4DY
Tel: 0209-842449

Dr J E Davies
Manor Surgery
Chapel Street
Redruth
Cornwall
TR15 2BY
Tel: 0209-313313

Dr G B Hughes
Clinton Road Surgey
19 Clinton Road
Redruth
Cornwall
TR15 2LL
Tel: 0209-218686

REPTON

Health Centre
Askew Grove
Repton
Derbyshire
DE6 6SH
Tel: 0283-703318

RETFORD

The Bridgegate Surgery
43 Bridgegate
Retford
Nottinghamshire
DN22 7UX
Tel: 0777-702381

Dr M J H B Waas
The Surgery
Sturton Road
North Leverton
Retford
Nottinghamshire
DN22 0AB
Tel: 0427-880223

RIBBLETON

Dr R T Parry
The Surgery
51 Longridge Road
Ribbleton
Preston
Lancashire
PR2 6RE
Tel: 0772-792512

RICKMANSWORTH

Gade House Surgery
99B Uxbridge Road
Rickmansworth
Hertfordshire
WD3 2DJ
Tel: 0923-775291

RICHMOND

The Clinic
King's Road
Richmond
Surrey
TW10 6EF
Tel: 081-940 9879

Dr G Ezekiel
The Vineyard Surgery
35 The Vineyard
Richmond
Surrey
Tel: 081-9480404

Dr A C Snape
The Surgery
36 Pagoda Avenue
Richmond
Surrey
TW9 2HG
Tel: 081-948 4217

Dr A V Kirkbride
The Surgery
1 Kew Gardens Road
Surrey
TW9 3HH
Tel: 081-940 1812

RIPLEY

Dr J W Aspinall
The Surgery
1 Ivy Grove
Ripley
Derbyshire
DE5 3HN
Tel: 0773-745059

ROCHDALE

Edesfield Road Surgery
Cutgate
Rochdale
Lancashire
OL11 5AA
Tel: 0706-344044

Dr P Rowlands & Partners
Spotland Group Practice
55 Spotland Road
Rochdale
OL12 6PQ
Tel: 0706-44584

ROCHESTER

Health Centre
Gun Lane
Strood
Rochester
Kent
ME2 4UL
Tel: 0634-717755

Appendix 1

Dr J H Redman
The Surgery
1 The Esplanade
Rochester
Kent
ME1 1QE

ROMFORD

Dr M Feldman
Petersfield Surgery
70 Petersfield Avenue
Harold Hill
Romford
RM3 9PD
Tel: 04023-43956

ROMSEY

Dr P J Burrows
Abbey Mead Surgery
Romsey
Hapshire
SO51 8EN
Tel: 0703-512218

Dr P J White
Nightingale Surgery
Greatwell Drive
Romsey
Hapshire
SO51 7QN
Tel: 0794-511513

ROOS

Dr W J Isherwood
The Surgery
Rectory Road
Roos
North Humberside
HU12 0LA
Tel: 0964-527427

ROTHERHAM

Stag Medical Centre
162 Wickersley Road
Rotherham
Yorkshire
S60 4JW
Tel: 0709-379285

ROWLANDS CASTLE

Dr J R Harrison
The Surgery
12 The Green
Rowlands Castle
Hampshire
PO9 6BN
Tel: 0705-412846/7

RUDGWICK

Dr W J Jarratt
The Health Centre
Rudgwick
West Sussex
RH12 3HB
Tel: 0403-822103

RUGBY

Central Surgery
Corporation Street
Rugby
Warwickshire
CV21 3SP

Dr C Longbotham
The Health Centre
Horse Fair
Rugby
Staffordshire
WS15 2EL

ST ALBANS

Harvey House Surgery
13/15 Russell Avenue
St Albans
Hertfordshire
AL3 5HB

Dr K Lancer
Highfield Clinic
Highfield Lane
St Albans
Herts
AL4 0RJ

Dr J H Sterland
283 High Street
London Colney
St Albans
AL2 1EL
Tel: 0727 823245

ST ANNES-ON-SEA

The Surgery
47 St Andrews Road South
St Annes-on-Sea
Lancashire
FY8 1PZ

Dr M Atherton
The Surgery
17 Park Road
St Annes-on-Sea
Lancashire
FY8 1PW

ST HELENS

International Vaccination
    Centre
St Helens Hospital
Peasley Cross Wing
Marshalls Cross Road
St Helens
Merseyside
WA9 3DA

ST GERMANS

Dr J R A Moore
Quay Lane Surgery
Old Quay Lane
St Germans
PL12 5LH
Tel: 0503 30088

ST MARY CHURCH

Dr P R Densham
The Medical Centre
Fore Street
St Mary Church
Torquay
Devon
TQ1 4QX

SALFORD

Dr S Haber
University of Salford
250 Langworthy Road
Salford
Manchester
M6 5WW

SALISBURY

The Surgery
Park Road
Tisbury
Salisbury
Wilts
SP3 6FF

Dr P Claydon
The Surgery
Common Road
Whiteparish
Salisbury
SP5 2SO

Public Health Lab Service
Centre for Applied Micro-
    biology Research
Porton Down
Salisbury
Wiltshire

Harcourt Medical Centre
Crane Bridge Road
Salisbury
Wiltshire
SP2 7TD

Dr R Willis
The Surgery
Salisbury
Wiltshire
SP1 2PH

Dr K L Williams
The Health Centre
Wilton
Salisbury
Wiltshire
SP2 0HT

SALTASH

Dr R C Cook
Saltash Health Centre
Callington Road
Saltash
Cornwall
PL12 6DL

SALWICK

Dr R C Goodfellow
British Nuclear Fuels Plc
Medical Department
Springfield Works
Salwick
Preston
Lancashire
PR4 0XJ

SANDWICH

YFVC
The Kent Private Clinic
1 The Butchery
Sandwich
Kent
CT13 9DL

SAXILBY

Dr N D Chapman
The Surgery Glebe House
Church Road
Saxilby
Lincoln
Lincolnshire
LN1 2HJ

SCARBOROUGH

Scarborough Hospital
Scalby Road
Scarborough
North Yorkshire
YO12 6QL

SELBY

Dr J D Reid
The Surgery
4 Prak Street
Selby
North Yorkshire
YO8 0PW

Dr M E Williams
Abbey Yard
Selby
YO8 0PN

SELSDON

Dr A Trompetas
The Surgery
60 Sundale Avenue
Selsdon
Surrey
CR2 8RP

SETTLE

Townhead Surgeries
Settle
North Yorkshire
BD24 9JA

SEVENOAKS

Dr F D Higgs
Amherst Medical Centre
London Road
Sevenoaks
Kent
TN13 2JD

Town Medical Centre
25 London Road
Sevenoaks
Kent
TN13 1AR

SHEFFIELD

Dr P R Allamby
2 Gomersal Lane
Dronfield
Sheffield
S18 6RU
Tel: 0246 290120

The Surgery
Mulberry Street
Sheffield
South Yorkshire
S1 2PL

Dr Kirersley
Richmond Medical Centre
334 Richmond Road
Sheffield
South Yorkshire
S13 8LY

Dr C Kell
The Practice
394 London Road
Sheffield
South Yorkshire
S2 4NB

Pharmacy Department
Middlewood Hospital
Sheffield
South Yorkshire
S6 1TP

Dr D A Keating & Partner
The Surgery
104 Elm Lane
Sheffield
South Yorkshire
S5 7TW

University Health Service
2 Claremont Place
Sheffield
South Yorkshire
S10 2TB

Dr I D Cooke
AMI Thornbury Hospital
312 Fulwood Road
Sheffield
South Yorkshire
S10 3RS

Dr D A Keating
11 Ecclesfield Road
Chapeltown
Sheffield
Yorkshire
S30 4TD

Dr R U Watson
Swallownext Health Centre
Hepworth Drive
Aston
Sheffield
Yorkshire
S31 0BG

Dr C S Barclay
The Nethergreen Surgery
34-36 Nethergreen Road
Sheffield
South Yorkshire
S11 1NG

Dr D G Morgan
Occupational Medical
    Services
The Coach House
16 Chapman Street
Sheffield
South Yorkshire
S9 1NG

Dr G N North
Shiregreen Medical Centre
492 Bellhouse Road
Sheffield
S5 0RG

Dr Sham Roop Lal Grover
The Surgery
899 Barnsley Road
Sheffield
South Yorkshire
S5 0QJ

Dr T S Singh
2 Harold Street
Sheffield
S6 3QB

The Surgery
British Airways Travel Clinic
Mount Avenue
Sheffield
ESSEX
CM13 2NL

SHENFIELD

BA Travel Centre
The Surgery
Mount Avenue
Shenfield
Essex
CM13 2NL

SHEPPERTON

Dr A Jones
Amey Medical Centre
Lee International Studies
Studio Road
Shepperton
Middlesex
TW7 0QD

Dr D J M Choat
Shepperton Health Centre
Shepperton Court
Laleham Road
Shepperton
Middlesex
TW17 8EJ

SHERBORNE

The Cross
Milborne Port
Sherborne
Dorset
DT9 5DH

SHERINGHAM

Dr Moss Taylor
Sheringham Medical Practice
The Health Centre
Sheringham
Norfolk
NR26 8RT

SHIFNAL

Dr M A Brinkley
Shifnal Medical Practice
Shrewsbury Road
Shifnal
Shropshire
TF1 8AJ

SHIPSTON-ON-STOUR

Dr P N Johnson
The Medical Centre
Badgers Crescent
Shipston-on-Stour
CV 36 4BQ

SHREWSBURY

Cross Houses Hospital
Shrewsbury
Shropshire
SY5 6JN

Dr E M Stapleton
Claremont Bank Surgery
Claremont Bank
Shrewsbury
Salop
SY1 1RL

The Pharmacy
Shrewsbury Hospital
Copthorne North
Mytton Oad Road
Shrewsbury
Shropshire
SY3 8YF

SIDCUP

Dr A K Carlile
Woodlands Surgery
146 HalfWay Street
Sidcup
Kent
DA15 8DF

SITTINGBOURNE

Dr E Mullard
Sidcup Health Centre
43 Granville Road
Sittingbourne
Kent
ME10 1ND

The Practice
32 London Road
Sittingbourne
Kent
ME10 1ND

SKEGNESS

Dr V J Rogers
4 Algitha Road
Skegness
Leicestershire
PE25 2AQ

SKIPTON

Dyneley House Surgery
Dyneley House
Newmarket Street
Skipton
Yorkshire
BD23 2HZ

The Practice
49 Otley Street
Skipton
Yorkshire
BD23 1ET

The Surgery
24/26 Main Street
Grassington
Skipton
Yorkshire
BD23 5AA

SLEAFORD

Sleaford Medical Group
Northgate
Sleaford
Lincolnshire
NG34 7BU

SLOUGH

The Nuffield Hospital
Wexham Street
Slough
Berkshire
SL3 6NH

Slough Occupational Health
    Service
30 Bradford Road
Buckingham Avenue
Slough
Berkshire
SL1 4PG

Windsor House
9 Albert Street
Slough
Berkshire
BL1 2BH

Dr R D Jones
Corporate Health Lrd
30 Bradford Road
Slough
Berkshire
SL1 4PG

Dr M S Dhatt
Langley Health Centre
Common Road
Langley
Slough
Berkshire
SL3 8LE

SOHAM

The Staploe Medical Centre
Brewhouse Lane
Soham
Cambridgeshire
CQ7 5JD

SOLIHULL

Dr S M Cowles
The Surgery
30 Winchcombe Road
Solihull
West Midlands
B92 8PJ

The Surgery
287 Haslucks Green Road
Shirley
Solihull
West Midlands
B90 2LW

Dr R E Nicol
Lapworth Surgery
Old Warwick Road
Lapworth
Solihull
West Midlands
B94 6LH

Dr E Layton
Shirley Medical Centre
8 Union Road
Shirley
Solihull
West Midlands
B90 3DT

Dr C T Landey
Park Surgery
278 Stratford Road
Shirley
Solihull
B90 3AF

Monkspath Surgery
Farmhouse Way
Shirley
Solihull
West Midlands
B90 4EH

Dr R H Morgan
1500 Warwick Road
Knowle
Solihull
West Midlands

Dr R E Nicol
3 The Avenue
Dorridge
Solihull
West Midlands
B93 8LH

Dr P J M Sloan
The Surgery
287 Haslucks Green Road
Shirley
Solihull
B90 2LW

Dr J L Robson
Medical Centre
100 Yew Tree Mane
Solihull
West Midlands
B91 2RA

SOMPTING

Dr W Ferguson
Ball Tree Surgery
Western Road North
Sompting
BN15 9UX

SONNING COMMON

Sonning Common Health
    Centre
Wood Lane
Sonning Common
Reading
Berkshire
RG4 9SW

SOUTH BRETTON

Dr A E Price
Screening Department
Fitzwilliam Hospital
Milton Way
South Bretton
Peterborough
PE3 8YQ

SOUTH CROYDON

Dr C Sudhakar
1 St Augustines Avenue
South Croydon
Surrey
CR2 6BA

Dr R D S Sanderson
The Surgery
53 Farley Road
Selsdon
South Croydon
CR2 7NG

Dr A Trumpetos
60 Sundale Avenue
Selsdon
South Croydon
Surrey
CR2 8RP

SOUTH HUMBERSIDE

Dr G P Kapil
20 Detuyll Street
Scunthorpe
South Humberside
DN15 7LS

SOUTH MIMMS

National Institute for
    Biological Standards and
    Control
South Mimms
Hertfordshire
EN6 3PG

SOUTHALL

Dr S W Rahman
Health Promotion Centre
57 Lady Margaret Road
Southall
Middlesex
UB1 2PH

Dr D J Mendle
1 Crosslands Avenue
Norwood Green
Southall
Middlesex
UB2 5QY

The Surgery
23 Beaconsfield Road
Southall
Middlesex
UB1 1BW

Dr M Garg
Allenby Travel Clinic
423 Allenby Road
Southall
Middlesex
UB1 2HG

SOUTHAMPTON

Cunard Steamship Company
Plc
South Western Houses
Canute Road
Southampton
Hampshire
SO9 1ZA

Dr R M Roope
51 Locks Road
Locks Heath
Southampton
SO3 6ZH

General Council of British
Shipping
19-23 Canute Road
Southampton
Hampshire
SO1 1FJ

Central Health Clinic
East Park Terrace
Southampton
Hampshire
SO9 4WA

The Aldermoor Health Centre
Aldermoor Close
Southampton
Hampshire
SO1 6ST

Shirley Health Centre
Grove Road
Shirley
Southampton
SO9 3ZZ

PPP Southampton Medical
Centre
PPP House
37 Commercial Road
Southampton
Hampshire
SO1 0GG

Dr W S Fleming
Fleet Medical Officer
P & O Lines Limited
Medical Department
Dukes Keep, Marsh LN
Southampton
SO9 4GU

The Pharmacy Store
Southampton General
Hospital
Tremona Road
Southampton
Hampshire
SO9 4XY

Dr C E Ursell
University Health Centre
The University
Highfield
Southampton
Hampshire
SO9 5NH

Dr D J Paynton
Bath Lodge Practice
Bittevue Health Centre
Commercial Road
Bittevue
Southampton, Hants
SO9 2DA

The Practice
2 Oxford Street
Southampton
Hampshire
SO1 1DJ

Dr N Evans
The Surgery
Lower Lane
Bishop's Waltham
Southampton
SO3 1GR
Tel: 0489 892288

Dr M Munro
Totton Health Centre
Testwood Lane
Southampton
SO4 3ZN
Tel: 0703 865051

SOUTHBOURNE

Southbourne Surgery
337 Main Road
Southbourne
Emsworth
Hants
P10 8JH

SOUTHEND-ON-SEA

Queensway Health Centre
PO Box 26
Queensway House
Essex Street
Southend-on-Sea
SS2 5TD

SOUTHPORT

Dr K R Nai Doo
The Surgery
107 Liverpool Street
Birkdale
Southport
Merseyside
PR8 4DB

Dr S J Bonnet
The Surgery
66 Station Road
Ainsdale
Southport
Merseyside
PR8 3HW

SOUTHSEA

The Surgery
23 Landport Terrace
Southsea
Hampshire
PO1 2RG

Dr J B Bennett
Somerstown Health Centre
Blackfriars Close
Southsea
Hampshire
PO5 4NJ

The Surgery
25 Osborne Road
Southsea
Hampshire
PO5 3ND

SOUTH SHIELDS

General Council of British
Shipping
4 Coronation Street
South Shields
Tyne & Wear
NE33 1AR

SOUTHWELL

Dr M S Duffy
The Health Centre
Burbage Green
Southwell
Nottinghamshire
NG25 OEW

SOUTHWICK

Dr R Titley
The Surgery
20 Southwick Street
Southwick
West Sussex
BN4 4TE

SOUTH WOOTON

Dr J E Burgess
Anglian Medical Services
17 Knight's Hall Village
South Wooton
Norfolk
PE30 3HQ

SPALDING

The Surgery
Moulton
Spalding
Lincolnshire
PE12 6NR

Dr C P Lemmon
High Street Surgery
15a High Street
Spalding
Lincolnshire
PE11 1TK

Dr D J Corlett
Church Street Surgery
Spalding
Lincolnshire
PE11 2PB

STAFFORD

The Surgery
13 Wolverhampton Road
Stafford
Staffordshire
ST17 4BP

Dr I M Turner
The Surgery
Sandy Lane
Brewood
Stafford
ST19 9ES

STAINES

Staines Private Medical
    Centre
10A Gorings Square
Church Street
Staines
Middlesex
TW18 4EP

STAMFORD

The Sheepmarket Surgery
Stamford
Lincolnshire
PE9 2SL

STANMORE

Dr G R Segal
Stanmore Surgery
9 Church Road
Stanmore
HA7 4AR

STANFORD LE HOPE

Dr S E Barton
The Surgery
37 Southend Road
Stanford Le Hope
Essex
SS17 0PQ

STANSTED

The Surgery
Redlands
86 St John's Road
Stansted
Essex
CM24 8JS

Dr J P G Spencer
British Airports Authority
Stansted Airport Ltd
Stansted
Essex
CM24 1QW

STEVENAGE

The Health Centre
5 Stanmore Road
Stevenage
Hertfordshire
SG1 3QA

Dr M Duggan
Manor House Surgery
Boxfield Green
Stevenage
Hertfordshire
SG2 7DS

STOCKBRIDGE

Dr D C Simpson
The Surgery
New Street
Stockbridge
Hampshire
SO20 6HG

STOCKFIELD

Dr D P Feeney
Branch End Surgery
Stockfield

STOCKPORT

Dr D J Riddell
Goyt Valley Medical Centre
Chapel Street
Whaley Bridge
Stockport
Cheshire
SK12 7BL

Dr D Dawson
Heaton Moor Health Centre
32 Heaton Moor Road
Stockport
Cheshire
SK4 4HX

Dr R Reisler
British Aerospace (C A) LTD
Chester Row
Woodford
Stockport
Cheshire
SK7 1QR

Dr Hany H Azmy
The Surgery
30 Brinnington Road
Stockport
Cheshire
SK1 2EX

Drs I D F Morgan & R S Briggs
The Health Centre
Chichester Road
Romiley
Stockport
Cheshire

Dr P L Harrison
Stockport Road Medical
    Practice
Marple
Stockport
Cheshire
SK6 6AB

Dr Judith A French
The Surgery
Town Street
Marple Bridge
Stockport
Cheshire
SK6 5AA

Heaton Moor Health Centre
32 Heaton Moor Road
Stockport
Cheshire
SK4 4NX

Dr G Brodie
The Health Centre
Thornbrook Road
Chapel-en-Le-Frith
Stockport
Cheshire
SL12 6LT

STOCKTON

Dr P Fletcher
Lawson Street Health Centre
Stockton
Cleveland
TS18 1HU

STOCKTON-ON-TEES

Dr R S Sagoo
Tennant Street Surgery
Stockton-on-Tees
Cleveland
TS18 2AT

Dr R A Douglass
Health Centre
Lawson Street
Stockton-on-Tees
Cleveland
TS18 1HX

STOKE POGES

British Airways Travel Clinic
Pavilion Clinic
Stoke Poges
Buckinghamshire
SL2 4JN

STOKE-ON-TRENT

Birches Medical Centre
Diana Road
Birches Head
Stoke-on-Trent
Staffordshire
ST1 6RS

Dr D L Colwell
Werrington Village Surgery
Ash Bank Road
Werrington
Stoke-on-Trent
Staffordshire
ST9 OJS

STOURBRIDGE

Dr S D Kelly
Worcester Street Surgery
24 Worcester Street
Stourbridge
West Midlands
DY8 1AW

STRATFORD-UPON-AVON

British Airways Travel Clinic
Rother House Medical Centre
Alcester Road
Stratford-Upon-Avon
Warwickshire
CV37 6PP

Dr N A Woodward
Bridge House Medical Centre
Scholars Lane
Stratford-on-Avon
Warwickshire
CV37 6HE

STROOD

Dr S C Davoodbhoy
St Mary's Medical Centre
Vicarage Road
Strood
Kent
ME2 4DG

STROUD

Dr R H Stephensom
The Health Centre
Beeches Green
Stroud
Gloustershire
GL5 4BH

STURMINSTER

The Surgery
Stalbridge
Sturminster Newton
Dorset
DT10 2RG

SUDBURY

Dr A Kemp
Siam Surgery
Sudbury
Suffolk
CO10 6JH

SUNBURY-ON-THAMES

International Medicine
UNOCAL Corporation
32 Cadbury Road
Sunbury-on-Thames
Middlesex
TW16 7LU

Dr S A F Helps
BP Research
Sunbury Research Centre
Chertsey Road
Sunbury-on-Thames
TW16 7LN

SUNNINGDALE

Dr J McKendrick
Magnolia House
Sunningdale
Berkshire
SL5 OQT

SUNNINGHILL

Dr P N Whitfield
Kings Corner Surgery
Sunninghill
Ascot
Berkshire
SL5 OAE

SURBITON

Dr C A Barlin
Berrylands Surgery
Howard Road
Surbiton
Surrey
KT5 8SA

Dr C A Aldous
317 Ewell Road
Surbiton
Surrey
KT6 7BX

SUTTON

Dr Latham
The Surgery
54 Ben Hill Avenue
Sutton
Surrey
SM1 4EB

Chief Pharmacist, JFVC
St Anthony's Hospital
London Road
Sutton
Surrey
SM3 9DW

SOUTH WIRRAL

Group Practice Centre
Old Chester Road
South Wirral
L66 3PB

SOUTH COLDFIELD

Dr C R M Broomhead
The Hanthorns Surgery
331 Birmingham Road
Sutton Coldfield
West Midlands
B72 1DL

SWANLEY

Dr W R Rumfeld
The Cedars Swanley
26 Swanley Centre
Swanley
Kent
BR8 7AH

SWANAGE

Dr R W Baker
The Health Centre
Station Approach
Swanage
Dorset
BH19 1HB

SWINDON

Dr N J A Theobald
Merchiston
10 Swindon Road
Stratton St Margaret
Swindon
Wiltshire
SN3 4QB

Swindon Private Health
    Centre
3 Cricklade Court
Swindon
Wiltshire
SN1 3EY

YFVC, Central Services Dept
Burmah Castrol UK Limited
Burmah House
Pipers Way
Swindon
Wiltshire
SN3 1RE

Old Court Surgery
Station Road
Wootton Bassett
Swindon
Wiltshire
SN4 7DZ

TADLEY

Holmwood Health Centre
Franklin Avenue
Tadley
Hampshire
RG26 6ER

TADWORTH

Dr Orme-Smith
Heathcote Medical Centre
Heathcote
Tadworth
Surrey
KT20 5TH

TAMWORTH

Dr P Ballard
The Aldergate Medical Centre
The Mount
Salters Lane
Tamworth
Staffordshire
B79 8BH

TAUNTON

District Headquarters
Wellsprings Road
Taunton
Devon
TA2 7PQ

Dr J Bowthorpe
Medical Centre
Creech St Michael
Taunton
Somerset
TA3 5QO

TEIGNMOUTH

Dr R N Gale
Channel View Surgery
Courtenay Place
Teignmouth
Devon
TW14 8AY

TELFORD

Charlton Medical Practice
Charlton Street
Oakesgates
Telford
Shropshire

Hollinswood Surgery
Downmead
Hollingwood
Telford
Shropshire
TF3 2EN

Dr P Barnes
Telford & District
    Occupational
Health Service Ltd
Halesford 13
Telford
TF7 4QP

Dr A Smith
Dawley Medical Practices
Dawley
Telford
Shropshire
TF4 3AL

THAME

The Health Centre
East Street
Thame
Oxon
OX9 3JZ

THATCHAM

The Health Centre
Thatcham
Newbury
Berkshire
RG18 4HH

THAXTED

Dr J M Robinson
The Surgery
Margate Street
Thaxted
Essex
CM6 2QN

THEALE

Dr J R Bywater
The Surgery
51 Church Street
Theale
Berkshire
RG7 5BX

THIRSK

The Surgery
Picks Lane
Thirsk
North Yorkshire
YO7 1PT

The Health Centre
Thirsk
North Yorkshire
YO7 1LG

THORNTON CLEVELEYS

Dr R Moore
Thornton Medical Centre
Church Road
Thornton Cleveleys
Lancashire
FY5 2TZ

TILBURY

Dr B Dutta
The Surgery
57 Calcutta Road
Tilbury
Essex
RH18 7QZ

TIMPERLEY

Dr B Caplan
Timperley Health Centre
169 Grove Lane
Timperley
WA15 6PH

Dr C Westwood
Timperley Health Centre
169 Grove Lane
Timperley
Altrincham
Cheshire
WA15 6PH

Appendix 1

TISBURY

The Surgery
Park Road
Tisbury
Salisbury
Wiltshire
SP3 6FF

TONBRIDGE

Dr J M Hawkings
Warders Medical Centre
East Street
Tonbridge
Kent
TN9 1LA

TORQUAY

Dr P R Densham
The Medical Centre
Fore Street
St Marychurch
Torquay
Devon
TQ1 4QX

TOWCESTER

Towcester Medical Centre
Link Way
Towcester
Northamptonshire
NN12 7HH

TRING

The Surgery
Rotheschild House
Chapel Street
Tring
Hertfordshire
HP23 6PU

TROWBRIDGE

Dr M Duckworth
Lovemead Group Practice
11 The Halve
Trowbridge
Wiltshire
BA14 8SH

TRURO

District Health Office
4 St Clements Vean
Tregolis Road
Truro
TR1 1NR

JFVC, Health Office
Cornwall & Isles of Scilly
AHA
The Leats
Truro
Cornwall
TR1 3AC

Royal Cornwall Hospital
Treliske
Truro
Cornwall
TR1 3LJ

Dr H M Dalal
18 Lemon Street
Truro
Cornwall
TR1 2LZ

TUNBRIDGE WELLS

Dr S A Hall
The Surgery
23 Upper Grosvenor Road
Tunbridge Wells
Kent
TN1 2DX

Dr A G Buckland
1st Floor Hill House
Clanricarde Road
Tunbridge Wells
Kent
TN1 1PJ

TWYFORD

The Surgery
Loddon Hall Road
Twyford
Berkshire
RG10 9JA

Dr J L O'Sullivan
Twyford Surgery
Hazeley Road
Twyford
Winchester
Hampshire
SO21 1QY

TYNE & WEAR

Dr K Overs
Palmer Community Hospital
Wear Street
Jarrow
Tyne & Wear
NE32 3UX
Tel: 091 489 7512

UCKFIELD

Dr Clive A Penketh
Uckfield Surgery
Uckfield
East Sussex
TN22 1EJ

ULVERSTON

Dr L A Wilson
Ulverstone Health Centre
Victoria Road
Ulverston
Cumbria
LA12 OEW
Tel: 0229 52223

UPAVON

Dr P D Jenkins
The Surgery
Upavon
Pensey
Wiltshire
SN9 6DZ

UPHOLLAND

Hall Green Surgery
164 Ormskirk Road
Upholland
Lancashire
WN8 OAB

UPMINSTER

The Surgery
226 St Mary's Lane
Upminster
Essex
RM14 3DH

UTTOXETER

The Surgery
36 Balance Street
Uttoxeter
Staffordshire
ST4 8JG

UXBRIDGE

Dr Yvonne Hollis
15 Windsor Street
Uxbridge
Middlesex
UB8 1AB

Dr Seager
Rank Zerox UK Limited
Bridge House
Oxford Road
Uxbridge
Middlesex

Appendix 1

Dr S J A Mort
Conley Community Surgery
4A Church Road
Cowley
Uxbridge
Middlesex
UB8 3NA

Dr J P Keech
BP Engineering
Uxbridge One
1 Harefield Road
Uxbridge
Middlesex
UB8 1PD

Dr C I McDonald
BP Exploration Operating Co
4-5 Long Walk
Stockley Park
Uxbridge
Middlesex
UB11 1BP

Dr Murray McEwan
Uxbridge Health Centre
George Street
Uxbridge
Middlesex
UB8 1UB

Dr P J Ryan
Glaxo Pharmaceuticals UK Ltd
Occupational Health Dept
Stockley Park West
Uxbridge
Middx
UB11 1BT

Dr S Ash
Ealing Hospital Travel Clinic
Pasteur Suite
Ealing Hospital
Uxbridge Road
Middlesex
UB1 3HW

VERWOOD

Dr J M L Segal
Elim
54 Manor Road
Verwood
Dorset
BH31 6EA
Tel: 0202 825353

WADEBRIDGE

Dr J M Barker
Mayfield Surgery
Fernleigh Road
Wadebridge
Cornwall
PL27 7AY
Tel: 0208 812342

WAKEFIELD

Dr A J Kidd
Health Centre
Ramsey Crescent
Middlestown
Wakefield
Yorkshire
WF4 4QQ

WANTAGE

Dr G A Dinnis
Newbury Street Practice
Wantage H/C Centre
Garston Lane
Wantage
Oxfordshire
OX12 7AY

Research and Development
Centre
Metal Box Plc
Denchworth Road
Wantage
Oxfordshire
OX12 9BP

WALLASEY

Dr J P Kingsland
St Hilary Brow Practice
204 Wallasey Road
Wallasey
Merseyside

Dr S K Tandon
The Health Centre
71 Grove Road
Wallasey
Merseyside
L45 3HF

Dr S Rudnick
Health Centre
Field Road
Wallasey
Wirral
Merseyside
L45 5JP

WALLINGFORD

The Medical Centre
Reading Road
Wallingford
Oxfordshire
OX10 9DU

WALLINGTON

Dr A C Hillyard
Shotfield Health Centre
Shotfield
Wallington
Surrey
SM6 OHY

WALSALL

Dr O S Manocha
The Surgery
16 Lichfield Street
Walsall
West Midlands
WS1 1TT

Dr B A N Reid
Salters Meadow Centre
Chase Terrace
Walsall
West Midlands
WS7 8AQ

Dr W Wells
15 Northgate
Aldrige
Walsall
West Midlands
WS9 8QD

WALTON-ON-THAMES

The Health Centre
Rodney Road
Walton-on-Thames
Surrey
KT12 3LB

Dr M T Banham
Gort House Surgery
32 Hersham Road
Walton-on-Thames
Surrey
KT12 1JX

WARE

Dr I H Bridges
Church Street Surgery
St Mary's Courtyard
Church Street
Ware
Hertfordshire
SG12 9EG

WARRINGTON

Dr P J Banyard
Bewsey St Medical Centre
40/42 Bewsey Street
Warrington
Cheshire
WA2 7JE

Dr P Reynolds
260a Padgate Lane
Warrington
WA1 3DN
Tel: 0925 815333

WARLEY

Dr M M Khan
The Surgery
51a New Birmingham Road
Tividale
Warley
W Midlands
B69 2JG

WASHINGTON

Dr D MacDermid
Victoria Road Health Centre
Concord
Washington
Tyne & Wear
NE37 2PU

WATERINGBURY

Dr D T Forsythe
94 Bow Road
Wateringbury
Kent
ME18 5DS

WATFORD

Coach House Surgery
12 Park Avenue
Watford
Hertfordshire
WD1 7HP

Dr S C Robertson
Hertfordshire Health Clinic
Abbotts House
198 Lower High St
Watford
WD1 2AJ

Dr A P Jackson
Sheepcast Medical Centre
80 Sheepcot Lane
Garston
Watford
Hertfordshire
WD2 6EB

WEAVERHAM

Dr M B Llewellyn
Weaverham Surgery
Northwich Road
Weaverham
Cheshire

WARWICK

Dr S H Desborough
Hastings House
Wellesbourne
Warwick
CV35 9NF

WELLINGBOROUGH

Dr I F Wall
The Redwell Medical Centre
1 Turner Road
Wellingborough
Northamptonshire
NN8 4UT

WELLINGTON

Dr G J Scott
Luson Surgery
Fore Street
Wellington
Somerset
TA21 8AB

WELWYN GARDEN CITY

Group Practice
4 Hall Grove
Welwyn Garden City
Herts
AL7 4PL

Dr A Reed
Bridge Cottage
41 High Street
Welwyn
AL6 9EF

WEMBLEY

The Surgery
19 Lancelot Road
Wembley
Middlesex
HA0 2AL

The Surgery
267 Ealing Road
Wembley
Middlesex
HA0 1EU

Dr Ashley L Krotosky
One Stanley Medical Centre
1 Stanley Avenue
Wembley
Middlesex
HAO 4JF

Dr M Raichura
95 Grasmere Avenue
Wembley
Middlesex
HA9 8TF

Dr A R Patel
Preston Medical Centre
23 Preston Road
Wembley
HA9 8JZ

Dr L P Goodchild
The Surgery
1 Uxendon Crescent
Wembley
Middlesex
HA9 9TW

Dr P Brent
The Surgery
124 Harrow Road
Wembley
Middlesex
HA9 6QQ

WEST BROMWICH

Dr P Verow
Sandwell Health Authority
Occupational Health
30 Hallam Close
Hallam Street
West Bromwich
B71 4HU

Midlands Occupational
      Health Service Limited
53 Birmingham Road
West Bromwich
West Midlands
B70 1PX

WESTBURY

Dr M Gumbley
Eastleigh Surgery
Station Road
Westbury
Wiltshire
BA13 3JD

WEMBURY

Dr S G Bennett
The Surgery
51 Hawthorn Drive
Wembury
Plymouth
Devon
PL9 OBE

WEST HALLAM

West Hallam Medical Centre
The Dales
West Hallam
Derbyshire
DE7 6GR

WOLVERHAMPTON

Dr N I Smith
Bredon House Private Medical
321 Tettenhall Road
Wolverhampton
West Midlands
WV6 OJZ

WESTON-SUPER-MARE

Dr P Watkinson
New Court Surgery
39 Boulevard
Weston-Super-Mare
Avon
BS23 1PF

WESTGATE-ON-SEA

The Surgery
60 Westgate Bay Avenue
Westgate-on-Sea
Kent
CT8 8SN

WEST KIRBY

Dr I Entwistle
Consultation Suite
27 Banks Road
West Kirby
Wirral
Merseyside
L48 0RA

WEST MALLING

West Malling Group Practice
Milverton
116 High Street
West Malling
Kent
ME19 6NE

WEYBRIDGE

Weybridge Health Centre
Minorca Road
Weybridge
Surrey
KT13 8DU

WEYMOUTH

Cross Road Surgery
Cross Road
Weymouth
Dorset

WHEATLEY

Dr A R Harnden
The Surgery
114 Church Road
Wheatley
Oxon
OX9 1LU

WHELLEY

Occupational Health Centre
Whelley Hospital
Whelley
Wigan
Manchester
WN1 3YZ

WHITBY

Springvale Medical Centre
Whitby
North Yorkshire
YO21 1SD

WHITEHAVEN

Ann Burrow Thomas Health
  Centre
c/o West Cumberland
  Hospital
Pharmacy Department
Hensingham
Whitehaven
Cumbria
CA28 8JG

Dr S A Bagshaw
The Surgery
27 Church Street
Whitehaven
Cumbria
CA28 7EB

WHITLEY BAY

The Surgery
64 Marine Avenue
Whitley Bay
Tyne & Wear
NE26 1NH

Dr J M Tose
Health Centre
Whitley Road
Whitley Bay
Tyne & Wear
NE26 2ND

WHITTLESEY

Dr A A Anderson
Jenner Health Centre
Turners Lane
Whittlesey
Cambridgeshire
PE7 4EJ

WICKHAM

Dr J F Bostock
Wickham Group Practice
Station Road
Wickham
Hampshire
PO11 5JL

WIGAN

Dr P J Southern
The Surgery
Dicconson Terrace
Wigan
Manchester
WN1 2AF

Dr P R Kreppel
Mesnes View Surgery
Mesnes Street
Wigan
WN1 1ST

Occupational Health Centre
Whelley Hospital
Bradshaw Street
Whelley
Wigan
Manchester
WN1 3UZ

WIGTON

Dr E Roderick
The Surgery
Caldbeck
Wigton
Cumbria
CA7 8DS

WILLENHALL

The Surgery
Ednam Hall
63 Bloxwich Road
Willenhall
West Midlands
WV13 1A

Dr A R Shah
66 Cannock Road
New Invention
Willenhall
West Midlands
WV12 5RZ

WILLITON

Dr W N Kingsbury
Williton Surgery
Williton
Taunton
TA4 4QE

WILMSLOW

Dr I G Donnon
MSF Aviation Ltd
Manchester Airport
Wilmslow
Cheshire
SK9 4LL

Dr J H Ainsworth
Westgate Surgery
75 Alderley Road
Wilmslow
Cheshire
SK9 1PA

WIMBORNE

Dr Timberlake & Dr M
   Blackmore
Heathlands House
175 Station Road
West Moors
Wimborne
Dorset
BH22 OHX

Dr D L Brown
Walford Mill Medical Centre
Knobcrook Road
Wimborne
Dorset
BH21 1NL

WINCHESTER

Dr J M Fowler
The Sarum Road Nursing
   Road
Sarum Road
Winchester
Hertfordshire

Dr K E Roberts
St Clement's Surgery
Tanner Street
Winchester
Hampshire
SO23 8AD

WINDSOR

Dr B Barua
Lee House
84 Osborne Road
Windsor
Berkshire
SL4 3EW

Dr R K Goulds
The Surgery
21 Sheet Street
Windsor
Berkshire
SL4 1BZ

OLD WINDSOR

Newton Court Medical Centre
Burfield Road
Old Windsor
Berkshire
S14 2QF

WINSFORD

Dr V Prasad
Swanlow Lane
Winsford
Cheshire
CW7 1JF

WING

Dr J A Lilley
The Surgery
46 Stewkley Road
Wing
Nr Leighton Buzzard
Bedfordshire
LU7 ONE

WINSLOW

Dr W I C Clark
The Surgery
24 Ham Street
Winslow
Buckinghamshire
MK18 3AL

Norden House Surgery
Avenue Road
Winslow
Buckinghamshire
MK18 3DW

WIRKWORTH

Dr A R Lindop
The Wirksworth Health
   Centre
St John Street
Wirkworth
Derbyshire
DE4 4DR

WISBECH

The North Brink Practice
7 North Brink
Wisbech
Cambs
PE13 1JU

Clarkson Surgery
De Havilland Road
Wisbech
Cambs
PE13 3AN

Dr J M Neary
Trinity Surgery
Norwich Road
Wisbech
Cambridgeshire
PE13 3UZ

WITLEY

Dr P R Wilks
Witley Surgery
Wheeler Lane
Witley
Surrey
GU8 5QR

WITHINGTON

Dr W P Tamkin
32 Burton Road
Withington
M20 9EB

WITNEY

Dr C A Lole-Harris
Windrush Practice
Windrush Health Centre
Witney
Oxfordshire
OX8 7HS

Nuffield Health Centre
Welch Way
Witney
Oxfordshire
OX8 7HA

WOKING

The Health Centre
Hermitage Road
St Johns
Woking
Surrey
GU21 1TD

Phillips Quadrant
35 Guildford Road
Woking
Surrey
GU22 7QT

Goldsworth Park Health
   Centre
Denton Way
Goldsworth Park
Woking
Surrey
GU21 3LO

Dr D J Williams
York House Medical Centre
Heathside Road
Woking
Surrey
GU22 7XL

WOLVERHAMPTON

Dr P Linnemann
The Surgery
80 Tettenhall Road
Wolverhampton
West Midlands
WM1 4TF

Bushbury Surgery
85 Northwood Park Road
Bushbury
Wolverhampton
WV10 8EY

WOODLEY

The Loddon Vale Practice
Hurricane Way
Woodley
Reading
Berkshire
RG5 4UX

WOODSTOCK

The Surgery
Park Lane
Woodstock
Oxfordshire
OX7 1UD

WORCESTER PARK

The Clinic
Manor Drive
Worcester Park
Surrey
KT4 7LG

WORCESTER

St John's House Surgery
28 Bromyard Road
St John's
Worcester
Herefordshire
WR2 5BY

Dr R A Cooke
Dept of Occupational Health
Worcester Royal Infirmary
Ronkswood Branch
Newton Road
Worcester
WR5 1JP

WORKINGTON

Ann Burrow Thomas Health
    Centre
South William Street
Workington
Cumbria
CA14 2ED

WORKSOP

Dr F J Hobson
Health Centre
Newgate Street
Worksop
Nottinghamshire
S80 1HP

WORPLESDON

Dr Hilary Trigg
Fairlands Surgery
21 Fairlands Road
Worplesdon
Surrey
GU3 3JB

WYE

Wye Surgery
Oxen Turn Road
Wye
Kent
TN25 5AY

WYLAM

Dr C J Roberts
The Surgery
51 Woodcraft Road
Wylam
Northumberland
NE41 8DH

YEOVIL

Hendford Wing
Hendford Surgery
74 Hendford
Yeovil
Somerset
BA20 1UJ

YORK

Monkgate Health Centre
31 Monkgate
York
Yorkshire
YO3 7PV

Dr M Barry
British Airways Travel Clinic
Priory Medical Centre
Cornlands Road
Acomb
York
YO2 3DS

Dr A L Harris
Haxby Health Centre
Haxby
York
Yorkshire
YO3 3PL

SCOTLAND

ABERDEEN

OMS
12 Sunnybank Road
Aberdeen
AB2 3NG
Tel: 0224-492884

View Terrace Clinic
1 View Terrace
Aberdeen
AB2 4RS
Tel: 0224-631633

Aberdeen Medical Services
Aberdeen Health Screening
    Clinic
6 Rubislaw Terrace
Aberdeen
AB1 1XE

Elmbank Group
Foresterhill H/C
Westburn Road
Aberdeen
AB9 2AY
Tel: 0224-696949

Gilbert Road Medical Group
39 Gilbert Road
Bucksburn
Aberdeen
AB2 9AW
Tel: 0224-712138

Foresterhill Health Centre
Suite A
Westburn Road
Aberdeen
AB2 9AY
Tel: 0224-695949

Aberdeen Industrial Doctors
21 Albyn Place
Aberdeen
AB9 1RJ
Tel: 0224-572879

AIRDRIE

The Surgery
Lauchope Street
Chappelhall
Airdrie
Tel: 0236-762144

AYR

Medicayr
3 Barns Street
Ayr
KA7 1XB
Tel: 0292-281439

BANNOCKBURN

Health Services Clinic
Firs Entry
Bannockburn
FK7 0HW
Tel: 0786-813435

DUMFRIES

The Surgery
32 Main Street
New Abbey
Dumfries
DG2 8BY
Tel: 0387-85263

DUNDEE

King's Cross Hospital
Clepington Road
Dundee
DD3 8EA
Tel: 0382-876116 EXT.2157

The Surgery
15 Camperdown Street
Broughty Ferry
Dundee
DD5 3AA
Tel: 0382-78881

EDINBURGH

Drs Ryecroft & Lacey
The Surgery
84 Main Street
Davidsons Mains
Edinburgh
EH4 5AB
Tel: 031-3362291

The Surgery
15-17 Carlton Terrace
Edinburgh
EH7 5DD
Tel: 031-5572100

British Airways Travel Clinic
Lifewatch-Edinburgh
4 Drumsheugh Gardens
Edinburgh
EH3 7QJ
Tel: 031-2262794/5

ELGIN

Braco Lodge
42 Mayne Road
Elgin
Morayshire
Tel: 0343-542234

GLASGOW

CD(S)U
Immunisation Clinic
Ruchill Hospital
Glasgow
G20 9NB
Tel: 041-9467120 EXT.254

British Airways Travel Clinic
Lifewatch-Glasgow
5-6 Park Terrace
Glasgow
G3 6BY
Tel: 041-3328010

GCBS Doctors
Marine Medical Services
209 Govan Road
Glasgow
G51 1HJ
Tel: 041-4276886

20 Cochrane Street
Glasgow
G1 1HX
Tel: 041-2274411

Ruthergien Health Centre
130 Stonelaw Road
Ruthergien
Glasgow
G73 2PQ
Tel: 041 647 7171

GOUROCK

Gourock Health Centre
181 Shore Street
Gourock
Renfreshire
PA19 1AQ
Tel: 0475-34617

HAMILTON

The Surgery
74 Portland Place
Hamilton
ML3 7LA
Tel: 282184

HAWICK

Hawick Health Centre
Teviot Road
Hawick
TD9 9DT
Tel: 0450-72076

INVERNESS

Dr H I McNamara
The Crown Medical Practice
12 Crown Avenue
Inverness
IV2 3NF
Tel: 0463-710777

Dr R Miller
Riverside Medical Practice
Ballifeary Lane
Ness Walk
Inverness
IV3 5PW
Tel: 0463 233191

IRVINE

Ayrshire General Hospital
Irvine
KA12 8SS
Tel: 0294-7419

KILWINNING

Kilwinning Medical Practice
15 Almswall Road
Kilwinning
KA13 6BL
Tel: 0294-54591

LANARK

Health Centre
South Vennel
Lanark
Strathclyde
ML11 7JT
Tel: 0555-3005

MORAY

Forres Health Centre
Castlehill
Forres
Moray
IV36 1OQF
Tel: 0309-72221

OBAN

Esplanade Surgery
Oban Times Building
Oban
Argyll
PA34 5PU
Tel: 0631-63175

ORKNEY

Orkney Health Board
New Scapa Road
Kirkwall
Orkney
KW15 1BH
Tel: 0865-2763 EXT.257

Appendix 1

PAISLEY

Dr D B Winton
The Love Street Medical
    Centre
36 Love Street
Paisley
Scotland
PA3 2DY
Tel: 041-8893355

PERTH

Drumhar Health Centre
North Methven Street
Perth
PH1 5PD
Tel: 0738-27912

SHETLAND ISLES

Gilbert Bain Hospital
SHETLAND
SE1 0RB
Tel: 0595-5678

STENHOUSEMUIR

Tryst Medical Centre
431 King Street
Stenhousemuir
Stirlingshire
FK5 4HT
Tel: 0324-551555

STIRLING

Dr G Kyles
Viewfield Medical Centre
3 Viewfield Place
Stirling
Scotland
FK8 1NJ
Tel: 0786-72028

WALES

CARDIFF

BA Travel Clinic
Lansdowne Hospital
Sanatorium Road
Canton
Cardiff
Wales CF1 8UL
Tel: 0222-378534

The Surgery
350 Cyncoed Road
Cyncoped
Cardiff
CF2 6XH
Tel: 0222-76515

Dr R P Edwards
Brynderwen Surgery
Crickhowell Road
St Mellons
Cardiff
CF3 OEF
Tel: 0222-799921

Dr R P Edwards
Minster Surgery
Minster Road
Roath
Cardiff
CF2 5AS
Tel: 0222-473999

CARMARTHEN

Dr Brennan
Morfa Lane Surgery
Carmarthen
SA31 3AX
Tel: 0267-234774

Dr C L John
Furnace House Surgery
St Andrews Road
Carmarthen
SA31 1LW
Tel: 0267-236616

CWMBRAN

Oak Street Surgery
Cwmbran
Gwent
NP44 3LT
Tel: 06333-66719

GWYNEDD

Dr D H Lazarus
Bodreinallt Surgery
Conwy
Gwynedd
LL32 8AT
Tel: 0492-593385

The Clinic
Aford Angle
Llandudno
Gwynedd

Aberconwy Community
    Office
Llandudno
Gwynedd
LL30 1LB
Tel: 0492-860011

The Health Centre
Blaenau Ffestiniog
Gwynedd
LL41 3DW
Tel: 0766-830205

HAVORFORDWEST

Dr Reynolds
Community Health Clinic
Department of Occupational
    Health
Withybush General Hospital
Haverfordwest
S61 2PZ
Tel: 0437-773217

Community Health Clinic
Merlins Hill
Haverfordwest
Dyfed
SA61 1PG
Tel: 0437-67801 EXT.251

HERFORD

Dr P J Matthews
Morefield House
Herford

LLANGOLLAN

Llangollan Health Centre
Regent Street
Llangollan
Clwyd
LL20 8HL
Tel: 0978-860625

LLAY

Dr A P Taffinder
The Health Centre
Llay
Clwyd
LL12 0TR
Tel: 0978-832206

MID GLAMORGAN

Parc Canol Surgery
Central Park
Church Village
Mid Glamorgan
Tel: 0443-203414

The Health Centre
1 Portway
Porthcawl
Mid Glamorgan
CF36 3XB
Tel: 0656-772620

Dr Din
Troed-y-Bryn Surgery
Penyrheol
Caerphilly
Mid Glamorgan
Tel: 0222-886501

MOLD

Clwyd Health Authority
Preswylfa
Hendy Road
Mold
Clwyd
HC7 1PZ

NEWPORT (GWENT)

Dr C L Bassi
St Pauls Clinic
Palmyra Place
Newport
Gwent
Tel: 0633-266140

Dr N Rajan
The Surgery
East Avenue
Bedwas
Newport
Gwent
NP1 8AE
Tel: 0222-864989

Clytha Clinic
Clytha Park Road
Newport
Gwent
Tel: 0633-64011

PRESTATYN

Ystwyth Medical Group
19-21 Portland Street
Ffordd Pendyffryn
Prestatyn
Clwyd
Tel: 0745-886444

POWYS

Dr J Wynn-Jones
The Surgery
Well Street
Montgomery
Powys
SY1 7ER
Tel: 0686-668217

Dr C S Townsend
The Medical School
Salop Road
Welshpool
Powys
SY1 7ER
Tel: 0938-553118

Dr J R Waring
The War Memorial Health
    Centre
Beauford Street
Crickhowell
Powys
NP8 1AG
Tel: 0873-810255

PONTYCLUN

Dr C J L Morgan
Central Surgery
Clun Avenue
Pontyclun
Mid Glamorgan
CF7 9AG
Tel: 0443-222567

SOUTH GLAMORGAN

Dr E F Griffith
British Shipping Vaccination
    Centre
15-16 Station Road
Penarth
S Glamorgan
CF6 2EP
Tel: 0222-702301

High Street Surgery
37-39 High Street
Barry
South Glamorgan
CF6 8EB
Tel: 0446-733355

WEST GLAMORGAN

Dr G S Smith
Health Centre
Water Street
Port Talbot
West Glamorgan
SA12 6HR
Tel: 0639-890983

SWANSEA

Swansea Central Clinic
21 Orchard Street
Swansea
SA1 1PN
Tel: 0792-51591 EXT.303

WELSHPOOL

Dr C S Townsend
The Medical Centre
Salop Road
Welshpool
Powys
SY21 7ER

WREXHAM

Dr G M Clements
Wrexham Travel Clinic
Clwyd Health Authority
16 Grosvenor Road
Wrexham

Dr P Saul
The Clinic
Beech Avenue
Rhos
Wrexham
Clwyd
Tel: 0978-854955
LL14 1AA

Dr Y Singh
Hillcreast Medical Centre
86 Holt Road
Wrexham
Clwyd
LL13 8RG

Dr C D Shaw
Strathbone Surgery
28 Chester Road
Wrexham
Clwyd
LL11 2SA
Tel: 0978-352055

Health Centre
Gresford
Wrexham
Clwyd
Tel: 0978-356551

NORTHERN IRELAND

BALLYMENA

The Yellow Fever Vaccination
    Centre
51 Castle Street
Ballymena
Co Antrim
BT43 7BT
Tel: 0266 656324

Ballymena Health Centre
Cushendall Road
Ballymena
Co Antrim
BT19 6HQ
Tel: 0266 42181

BANGOR

Springhill Surgery
4A Killeen Avenue
Bangor
Co Down
BT19 1PP
Tel: 0247 472751

BELFAST

The Yellow Fever Vaccination
    Centre
The Clinic
Licoln Avenue
Belfast
Tel: 0232 748363

Dr Philip McCrea Associates
Moderna House
Quayside Office Park
Dargan Crescent
Belfast
BT3 9JP
Tel: 0232 370058

Limited access only:
University Health Service
The Queen's University of
    Belfast
Belfast
BT7 1NN
Tel: 0232 245133 Ext 3718

COOKSTOWN

The Oaks Family Medical
    Centre
48 Orritor Road
Cookstown
Co Tyrone
BT80 8BG
Tel: 0648 762249

DROMARA

The Surgery
Begny Hill Road
Dromara
Co Down
BT25 2AT
Tel: 0238 532217

FINTONA

Drs Sweeny, Magfhogartia,
    Monaghan
Fintona Medical Centre
Grianan
Carnalea Road
Fintona
Co Tyrone
BT78 2BY
Tel: 0622 841203

LIMAVADY

Drs Finlay, Campell,
    McQuillan
Bovally Medical Centre
Edenmore Road
Limavady
Co Londonderry
BT49 OTE
Tel: 0504 762321

OMAGH

The Yellow Fever Vaccination
    Centre
The Health Centre
Mountjoy Road
Omagh
Co Tyrone
Tel: 0662 243521 Ext 263

PORTADOWN

Portadown Health Centre
Tavanagh Avenue
Portadown
Craigavon
Co Armagh
BT62 3AJ
Tel: 0762 334400

JERSEY

Dr D Haydon Taylor
Lister House Surgery
The Parade
St Helier
Jersey
Channel Islands
Tel: 0534 36336

Dr S Slaffer
20 David Place
St Helier
Jersey
Channel Islands
Tel: 0534 20314

GUERNSEY

Dr C H White
Board of Health
Public Health Department
Lurkis House
Grange
Guernsey
Channel Islands

ISLE OF MAN

Noble's Hospital
Douglas
Isle of Man